SUPER**FOODS**

50 BEST FOODS TO CHANGE YOUR LIFE

This edition published by Parragon Books Ltd in 2014 and distributed by

Parragon Inc.
440 Park Avenue South, 13th Floor
New York, NY 10016
www.parragon.com/lovefood

LOVE FOOD is an imprint of Parragon Books Ltd

ISBN 978-1-4723-3248-6

Printed in China

Photography by Clive Streeter
Nutritional information by Judith Wills

Notes for the Reader
This book uses standard kitchen measuring spoons and cups. All spoon and cup measurements are level unless otherwise indicated. Unless otherwise stated, milk is assumed to be whole, eggs are large, individual vegetables are medium, and pepper is freshly ground black pepper. Unless otherwise stated, all root vegetables should be washed in plain water and peeled prior to using.

For best results, use a food thermometer when cooking meat and poultry. Check the latest USDA government guidelines for current advice.

Serving suggestions are all optional and not necessarily included in the recipe ingredients or method.

The times given are only an approximate guide. Preparation times differ according to the techniques used by different people and the cooking times may also vary from those given. Optional ingredients, variations, or serving suggestions have not been included in the time calculations.

Recipes using raw or very lightly cooked eggs should be avoided by infants, the elderly, pregnant women, convalescents, and anyone with a weakened immune system. Pregnant and breast-feeding women are advised to avoid eating peanuts and peanut products. People with nut allergies should be aware that some of the prepared ingredients used in the recipes in this book may contain nuts. Always check the packaging before use.

Vegetarians should be aware that some of the prepared ingredients used in the recipes in this book may contain animal products. Always check the package before use.

Picture acknowledgments
Cover images: Salad bowl with green salad © Creative Crop/Getty Images, Blueberries in cup © Getty Images/anna hwatz photography, Vegetables on cutting board © Getty Images/Scott & Zoe (also reproduced on page 3).

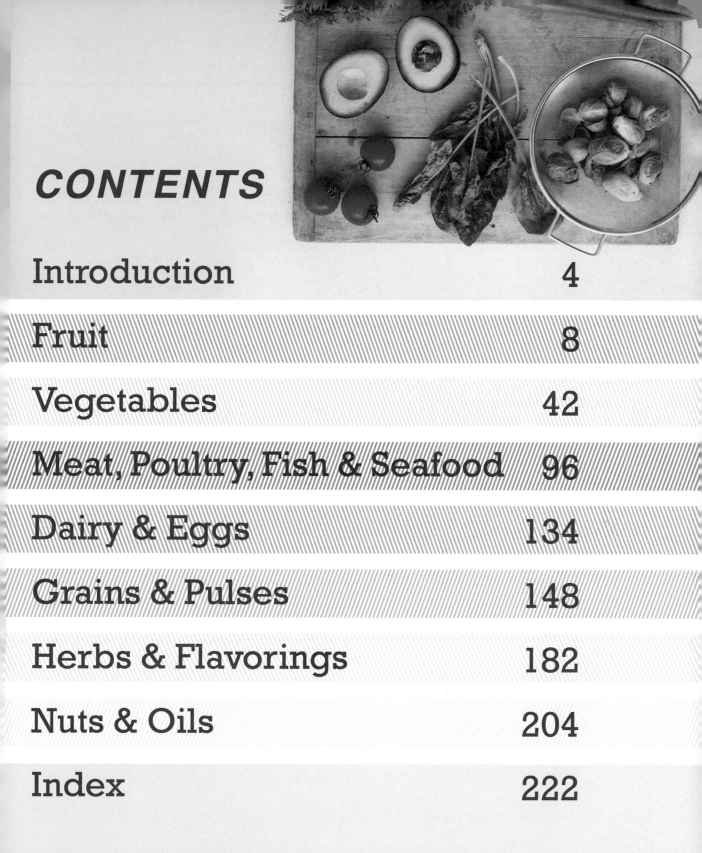

CONTENTS

INTRODUCTION

If you want to live a long and healthy life, there are many simple lifestyle changes that can boost both your brain and body functions. Most experts agree that the secret to a healthy lifestyle requires just a little common sense—clean living, eating a balanced diet, and getting plenty of exercise are all important. Choosing a healthy diet that is rich in superfoods is an easy step to improving how you look and feel.

What is a superfood?

The theory that certain foods can have a lasting effect on our health and well-being is certainly not a new one. More than two thousand years ago the father of modern medicine, Hippocrates, wrote about the link between diet and health, and modern-day physicians and dietitians are increasingly looking to our diet and so-called superfoods to help prevent and treat a whole host of diseases, including cancer, heart disease, Alzheimer's disease, stroke, cataracts, and many others.

All foods have some nutritional value, but superfoods earn their name because they contain particularly high levels of a particular vitamin, mineral, essential fatty acid, or phytochemical that has been shown to improve some aspect of our health or well-being.

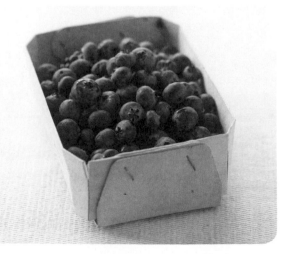

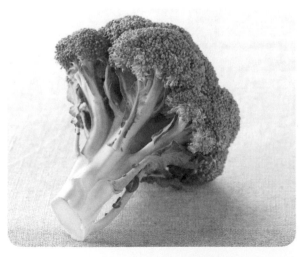

Superfoods come in all shapes and sizes, but the best way to be sure that you get a good selection is to make plant-based foods—such as fruit and vegetables, whole-grain cereals, beans, nuts, and seeds—the dominant ingredients in your diet.

In the pages that follow, you will find a whole host of superfoods that are readily available, easy to prepare, and make a delicious addition to your usual diet. Each page details the nutritional benefits that can be found in a particular ingredient, along with information on how best to prepare and store certain foods.

Superfood facts

• Some superfoods, such as blueberries, red bell pepper, and oranges, have vitamins and antioxidants that help reduce damage to cells.

• Green leafy vegetables, such as broccoli, kale, and watercress, contain naturally occurring plant chemicals, called phytochemicals, which work to block the growth of cancerous cells.

• Others, such as garlic and onions, earn their superfood status because they actively help to strengthen the immune system by boosting the body's natural resistance to disease and infection.

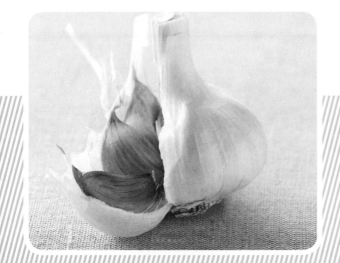

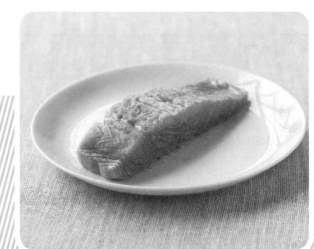

• Oil-rich fish, such as salmon, fresh tuna, mackerel, and sardines, offer a wealth of health benefits. The omega-3 fats found in these fish help to keep the heart healthy and also have an anti-inflammatory effect, which can help to relieve the symptoms associated with such conditions as rheumatoid arthritis.

• Studies have also shown that regular inclusion of oily fish in the diet can help improve concentration for both children and adults—and although they won't actually make you smarter, as many people believe, they certainly have a beneficial effect on mental focus and productive output.

• Many herbs and spices have superfood qualities. Cinnamon for instance, which is a key ingredient in many sweet recipes, is believed to help lower bad cholesterol and improve blood-sugar levels. It also has anti-inflammatory and antibacterial properties that help to fight infection in the body.

Choosing superfoods
The good news is that, despite their incredible health-boosting properties, superfoods don't have to be expensive or exotic—many of the fruits and vegetables we consume every day, such as carrots, beets, apples, lentils,

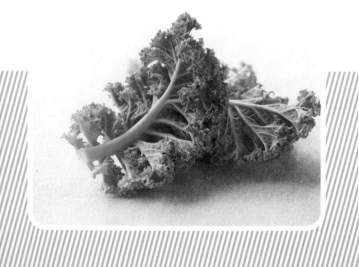

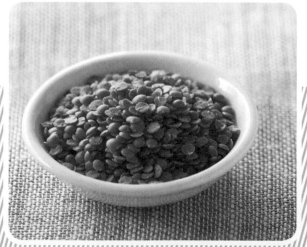

and tomatoes, contain compounds that technically make them superfoods. Put simply, this means that making the change to a healthy, balanced diet doesn't have to be expensive, and doesn't require hunting in health-food stores for unusual ingredients—just include more of the good stuff!

The theory that eating certain foods can help you live a longer and healthier life has been supported by a growing body of evidence from around the world. Some studies suggest that the right diet may even help counteract the negative effects of smoking, lack of exercise, and the stresses of modern living, and that certain foods could be the answer to niggling health problems such as indigestion, headaches, and lack of energy. It might seem as though the easy alternative to a diet overhaul is to take a vitamin pill every morning, but it's important to remember that most superfoods contain a cocktail of active ingredients and it's this combination (and interaction) that offers the health benefits.

In this book, we'll give you the lowdown on the top-50 everyday superfoods for you—and show you how to supercharge your diet with quick, easy, and delicious recipes packed full of goodness!

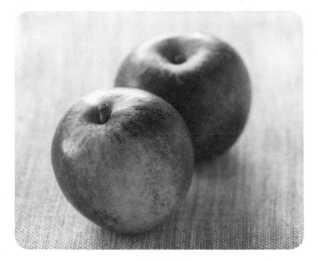

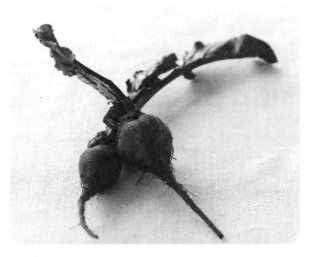

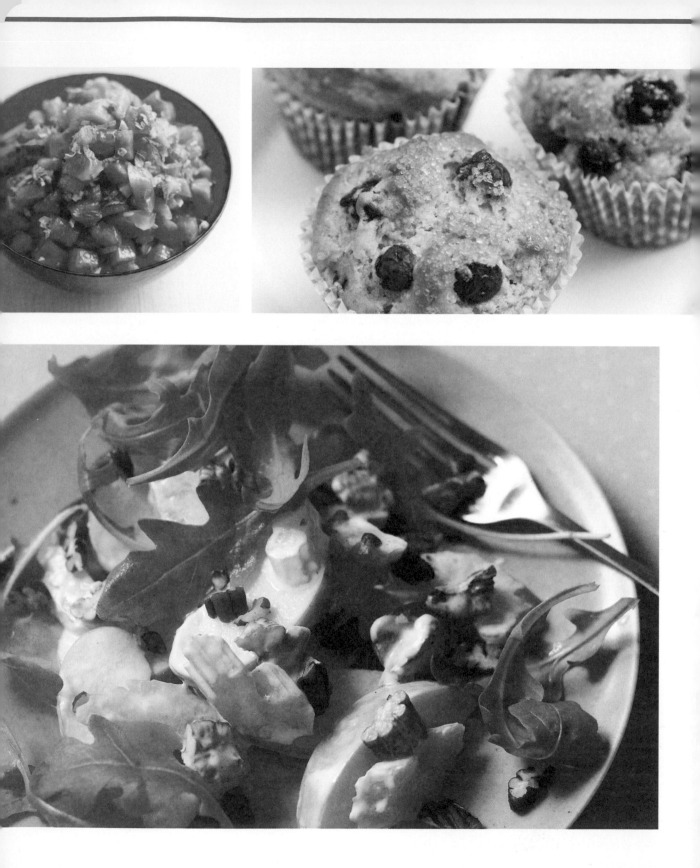

FRUIT

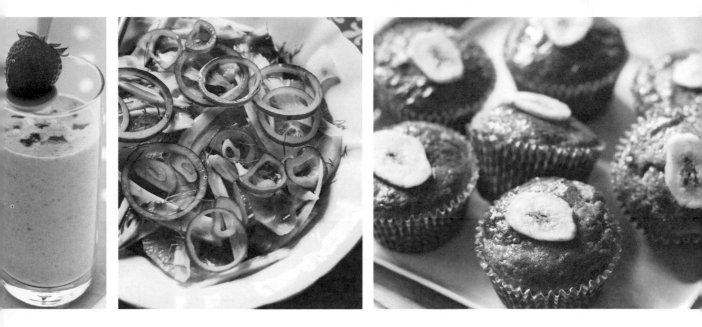

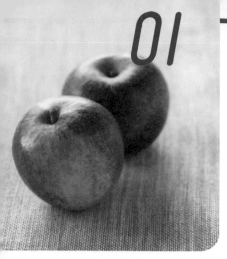

01

APPLES

In recent years, scientific evidence has shown that the old health proverb—an apple a day keeps the doctor away—may, in fact, be correct.

Although apples don't, with the exception of potassium, contain standout amounts of any particular vitamin or mineral, they do contain high levels of various plant chemicals, including the flavonoid quercetin. This is effective in protecting the body against a wide variety of diseases, including cancer and Alzheimer's, and it also has anti-inflammatory properties. Apples are a valuable source of pectin, a soluble fiber that can help to lower bad cholesterol (which can slowly build up in the inner walls of the arteries that feed the heart and brain) and help prevent colon cancer. Research has found that adults who regularly eat apples have smaller waistlines, less abdominal fat, and lower blood pressure than those who don't.

• Rich in flavonoids for healthy heart and lungs.
• Low in calories and low on the glycemic index (GI).
• High fiber content that is good for digestion.
• A good source of potassium, which can prevent fluid retention.

Practical tips:
Keep apples in a dark, cool place, such as your refrigerator, or a cupboard—they should be stored in a plastic bag with air holes in order to retain maximum amounts of their vitamin C content. To prevent browning, place cut slices into a bowl of water with 1–2 tablespoons of lemon juice. Always try to eat the skin because it contains up to five times as many plant chemicals as the flesh.

MAJOR NUTRIENTS PER AVERAGE APPLE

Calories	60
Total fat	trace
Protein	trace
Carbohydrate	16g
Fiber	2.8g
Vitamin C	5mg
Potassium	123mg

PORK CHOPS BRAISED WITH APPLES

SERVES 4

2 tablespoons olive oil
4 lean pork chops
12 small shallots, peeled
3 celery stalks, sliced
2 Pippin apples,
cored and sliced
1 cup chicken stock
2 tablespoons Worcestershire
sauce
1 tablespoon finely chopped
fresh rosemary
fresh rosemary sprigs,
to garnish

METHOD

1   Heat the oil in a large, wide saucepan or flameproof casserole dish, add the pork chops, and cook, turning once, for 2–3 minutes, until lightly browned.

2   Add the shallots and celery and cook for an additional 2 minutes, until lightly browned.

3   Stir in the apples, then add the stock, Worcestershire sauce, and chopped rosemary and bring to a boil. Reduce the heat to low, cover, and simmer gently for about 1 hour, until the meat is tender. To check when the pork is cooked, insert a meat thermometer into the thickest part of the meat; it should read at least 160°F. Or insert the tip of a sharp knife into the center of the meat and check that there is no pink meat and the juices are clear.

4   Garnish with rosemary sprigs and serve.

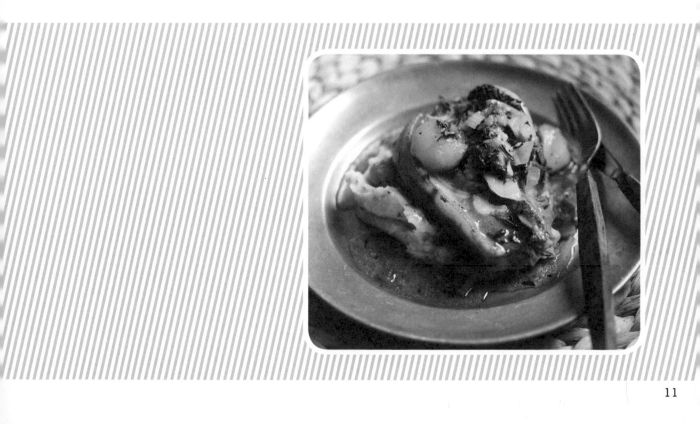

WALDORF SALAD

SERVES 4

½ cup pecans

4 apples, such as Cortland, Empire, or Red Delicious

juice of 1 lemon

4 celery stalks, thinly sliced

½ cup halved red seedless grapes

1 cup plain yogurt

4 cups arugula

pepper, to taste

METHOD

1   Toast the pecans in a skillet for a few minutes to bring out their flavor. When they are cool enough to handle, coarsely chop them.

2   Peel and chop the apples, then toss them in a bowl with the lemon juice to prevent them from discoloring.

3   Add the celery, grapes, and half the pecans to the apples and mix well. Stir in the yogurt and season with pepper, then gently toss together.

4   Divide the arugula among four serving plates and spoon over the salad mixture. Sprinkle the remaining nuts over the salad.

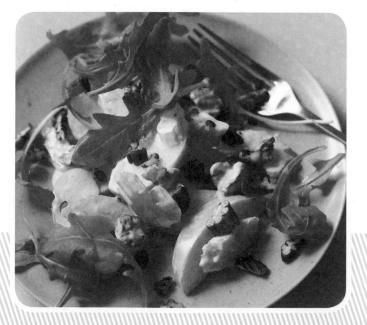

APPLE & CINNAMON BRAN MUFFINS

MAKES 12

¼ cup vegetable oil

1 tablespoon glycerin

¾ cup applesauce

2 eggs

½ teaspoon vanilla extract

¼ cup honey

¼ cup milk

2⅓ cups all-purpose flour

1¼ cups oat bran

⅔ cup ground flaxseed

1 teaspoon baking powder

½ teaspoon baking soda

½ teaspoon xanthan gum

1 teaspoon cinnamon

¼ teaspoon allspice

¾ cup firmly packed light brown sugar

¾ cup raisins

METHOD

1 Preheat the oven to 350°F. Line a 12-cup muffin pan with muffin cups.

2 In a large bowl, beat together the vegetable oil, glycerin, applesauce, eggs, vanilla extract, honey, and milk. In a separate bowl, mix together all the remaining ingredients, then add the liquid mixture and stir well.

3 Divide the batter among the muffin cups. Bake the muffins in the preheated oven for 20–25 minutes, or until a toothpick inserted into a muffin comes out clean. Remove from the oven and cool on a wire rack.

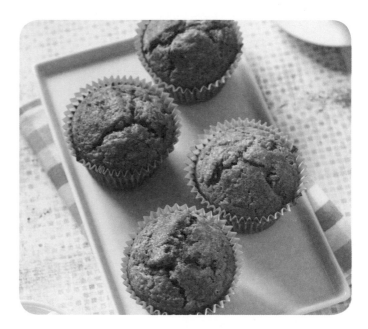

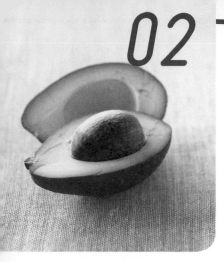

02

AVOCADOS

The buttery, green flesh of the avocado is a rich source of monounsaturated fats, which are important for a healthy heart, and it is packed with other important nutrients.

Avocados are high in fat, but this fat is mostly monounsaturated, which can, in fact, help to reduce bad blood cholesterol levels. The oleic acid contained in monounsaturates has also been linked with a lower risk of breast cancer. Avocados boast a large range of other nutrients, including vitamins C, E, and B6, folate, iron, magnesium, and potassium. They also contain the antioxidant plant chemical beta-sitosterol, which has been shown to improve blood cholesterol levels, help to prevent cancer, and has even been linked to improving age-related male hair loss.

- High vitamin E content boosts the immune system.
- Lutein helps protect against eye cataracts and age-related degeneration of the retina.
- High monounsaturated fat helps lower cholesterol.
- Good source of magnesium for a healthy heart.

Practical tips:
Choose avocados that have unblemished skins without soft spots, which suggest bruising. They're ready to eat if the flesh yields slightly when pressed with the thumb. To hasten ripening, put them in a paper bag with a banana. To prepare, cut lengthwise down to the pit and twist to separate the two halves. Pierce the pit with the tip of a knife, then pull to remove. Once cut, use lemon juice or vinegar to prevent discoloration.

MAJOR NUTRIENTS PER AVERAGE AVOCADO

Calories	240
Total fat	3g
Protein	2.2g
Carbohydrate	12.8g
Fiber	5g
Vitamin C	9mg
Potassium	728mg
Vitamin E	3mg

SPICY AVOCADO DIP

SERVES 4

2 large avocados

juice of 2 limes, or to taste

2 large garlic cloves, crushed

1 teaspoon mild chili powder, or to taste

salt and pepper, to taste

METHOD

1   Cut the avocados in half. Remove the pits and discard. Scoop out the flesh and discard the skins.

2   Place the avocado flesh in a food processor with the lime juice. Add the garlic and chili powder and process until smooth.

3   Transfer to a serving bowl, season with salt and pepper, and serve.

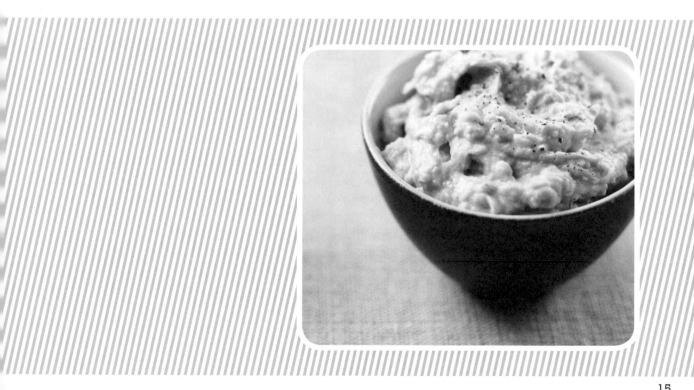

CHILLED AVOCADO SOUP

SERVES 4

2 avocados

1 tablespoon lemon juice

1 tablespoon snipped fresh
chives, plus extra to garnish

1 tablespoon chopped fresh
flat-leaf parsley

2 cups chicken stock, chilled

1¼ cups light cream,
plus extra to serve

dash of Worcestershire sauce

salt and pepper, to taste

METHOD

1   Halve the avocados and remove the pits. Scoop out the avocado
    flesh and coarsely chop.

2   Put the avocado, lemon juice, chives, parsley, stock, cream,
    and Worcestershire sauce in a blender or food processor and
    process until smooth. Season with salt and pepper.

3   Transfer the soup to a bowl, cover, and chill until required.
    Serve with light cream drizzled over the soup, topped with
    snipped chives.

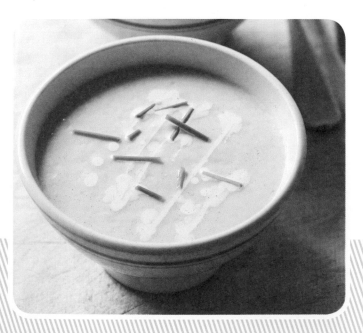

CITRUS-AVOCADO SALAD WITH HONEY DRESSING

SERVES 6

4 cups torn spinach leaves

4 cups torn romaine lettuce

1 cup torn iceberg lettuce

2 oranges, peeled and sectioned, membranes removed

1 grapefruit, peeled and sectioned, membranes removed

1 avocado, peeled, pitted, and sliced

1 tablespoon lemon juice

1 small onion, sliced

½ cup sliced celery

½ cup coarsely chopped pecans, toasted

HONEY DRESSING

⅓ cup sugar

2½ tablespoons lemon juice

2½ tablespoons honey

2 tablespoons cider vinegar

½ teaspoon dry mustard

½ teaspoon paprika

¼ teaspoon salt

⅛ teaspoon celery seeds

½ cup vegetable oil

METHOD

1 Combine the spinach, romaine, and iceberg lettuce in a large bowl. Arrange orange sections and grapefruit sections over the salad greens.

2 Toss the avocado slices gently with lemon juice, then discard the excess lemon juice. Arrange the avocado, onion, and celery over the salad. Sprinkle with pecans.

3 To make the honey dressing, combine all the ingredients, except the oil, in a food processor. Process until smooth. While the processor is running, slowly pour in the oil. Continue to process for a few seconds, until the oil is fully combined. Serve the salad drizzled with the dressing.

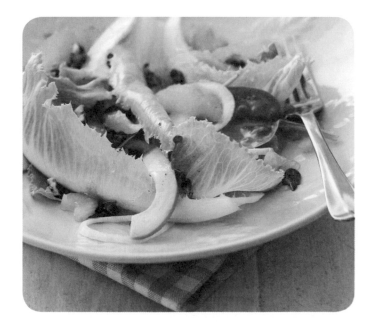

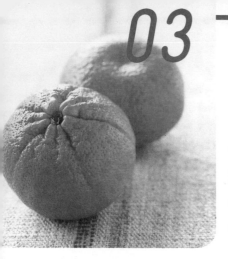

03

ORANGES

Vitamin C, the antioxidant vitamin that boosts the immune system and protects against the signs of aging, is found in abundance in oranges.

MAJOR NUTRIENTS PER AVERAGE ORANGE

Calories	65
Total fat	**Trace**
Protein	1g
Carbohydrate	16g
Fiber	3.4g
Vitamin C	64mg
Potassium	238mg
Calcium	61mg
Lutein/Zeaxanthin	182mcg

Oranges are one of the least expensive sources of vitamin C, which protects against cell damage and disease. The fruit is also a good source of fiber, folate, and potassium as well as calcium, which is vital for bone maintenance. They contain the carotenes zeaxanthin and lutein, both of which can help to maintain eye health and protect against degeneration of the retina. Oranges also contain rutin, a flavonoid that can help slow down or prevent the growth of tumors, and nobiletin, an anti-inflammatory compound. All these plant compounds also help the vitamin C in oranges work more effectively.

• High levels of vitamin C, which helps to prevent infections and reduce the severity and duration of colds.
• Low on the glycemic index (GI), so a useful fruit for dieters and diabetics.
• Good content of soluble fiber pectin, which helps control blood cholesterol levels.
• Anti-inflammatory, so may help reduce incidence of arthritis.

Practical tips:
Buy oranges that feel heavy to hold compared with their size—this means they should be juicy and fresh. Store them in the refrigerator to retain their vitamin C content. Orange peel contains high levels of nutrients, but should be scrubbed and dried before use.

DID YOU KNOW?

You should eat some of the white pith of the orange, as well as the juicy flesh, because it contains high levels of fiber, useful plant chemicals, and antioxidants.

ROAST SEA BASS WITH FENNEL & ORANGE

SERVES 2

12 ounces new potatoes, halved if large

2 tablespoons olive oil

1 small orange

2 whole sea bass, about 1 pound each, cleaned, scaled, and heads and fins removed

½ fennel bulb, thinly sliced

1 tablespoon roughly chopped fresh rosemary

1 tablespoon butter, melted

2 garlic cloves, thinly sliced

salt and pepper, to taste

METHOD

1   Preheat the oven to 400°F. Put the potatoes in a large roasting pan and drizzle with 1 tablespoon of the oil. Toss to coat, and roast in the preheated oven for 20 minutes.

2   Meanwhile, pare the zest from the orange using a zester. Cut the orange into slices. Make three or four cuts in the thickest part of each sea bass on both sides, cutting almost down to the bone. Season with salt and pepper and place two orange slices in the cavity of each.

3   Add the fennel and rosemary to the roasting pan. Toss with the potatoes and season with salt and pepper. Place the sea bass among the vegetables.

4   Mix together the orange zest, melted butter, garlic and remaining oil. Spoon over the sea bass. Scatter over the remaining orange slices, then return the roasting pan to the oven for a further 20 minutes, until the fish is just cooked through and the vegetables are tender. Serve immediately.

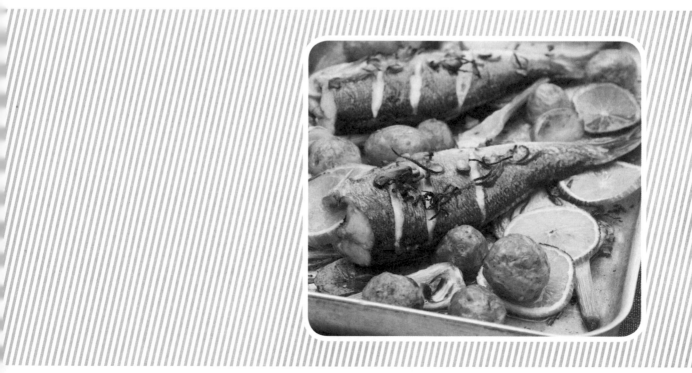

FENNEL SALAD

SERVES 4

2 oranges
1 bulb fennel, thinly sliced
1 red onion, sliced into
thin rings
pepper, to taste
fennel leaves, to garnish

DRESSING
juice of 1 orange
2 tablespoons balsamic
vinegar

METHOD

1 Peel and slice the oranges.
2 Arrange the orange slices in the bottom of a shallow dish.
Place a layer of fennel on top and then add a layer of onion.
3 To make the dressing, mix together the orange juice and
vinegar. Drizzle it over the salad. Season with pepper, garnish
with fennel leaves, and serve.

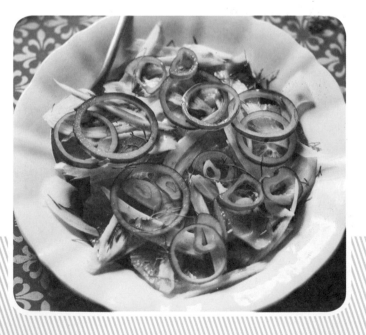

BROILED CINNAMON ORANGES

SERVES 4

4 large oranges
1 teaspoon ground cinnamon
1 tablespoon raw brown sugar

METHOD

1 Preheat the broiler to high. Cut the oranges in half and discard any seeds. Using a sharp knife, carefully cut the flesh away from the skin by cutting around the edge of the fruit. Cut across the segments to loosen the flesh into bite-size pieces that will then spoon out easily.

2 Arrange the orange halves, cut-side up, in a shallow, flameproof dish. Mix the cinnamon with the sugar in a small bowl and sprinkle evenly over the orange halves.

3 Cook under the preheated broiler for 3–5 minutes, until the sugar has caramelized and is golden and bubbling. Serve immediately.

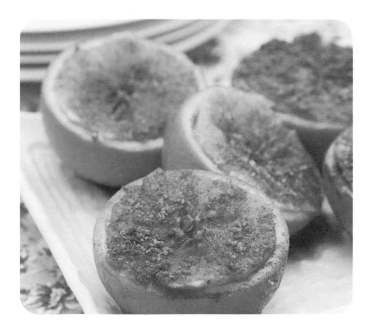

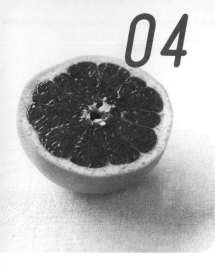

04

GRAPEFRUIT

The perfect healthy breakfast—the grapefruit, like many other citrus fruits, is an excellent source of vitamin C, which boosts the immune system.

In recent years, the pink-fleshed grapefruit has become as popular as the white or yellow-fleshed variety. It is a little sweeter and contains more health benefits—the pink pigment indicates the presence of lycopene, which has been shown to help prevent prostate and other cancers. Like other citrus fruits, the grapefruit contains bioflavonoids—compounds that appear to increase the benefits of vitamin C, which is also found in this fruit in excellent amounts. The grapefruit is low on the glycemic index (GI) and low in calories, so it is an important fruit for dieters. Because grapefruit juice can alter the effect of certain prescription medicines (such as those that lower blood pressure), people on medication should check with their physicians before they consume the fruit.

- High in antioxidants, which can help prevent prostate and other cancers.
- Rich in vitamin C to boost the immune system.
- Excellent fruit for dieters.

Practical tips:
Grapefruit is delicious halved, sprinkled with raw sugar, and broiled for a short while, and makes the perfect healthy breakfast. Always try to eat some of the white pith with your grapefruit, because this is also high in nutrients. Grapefruit, like all citrus fruits, will contain more juice if they feel heavy in relation to their size.

MAJOR NUTRIENTS PER HALF PINK GRAPEFRUIT

Calories	30
Total fat	Trace
Protein	0.5g
Carbohydrate	7.5g
Fiber	1.1g
Vitamin C	37mg
Potassium	127mg
Beta-carotene	770mcg
Folate	9mcg
Calcium	15mg

DID YOU KNOW?

The slightly bitter taste of some grapefruit is caused by a compound known as naringenin, which has cholesterol-lowering properties.

TROPICAL FRUIT SALSA

SERVES 4

1 small wedge watermelon, about 4 ounces

1 pink grapefruit

1–2 fresh green jalapeño peppers

2 teaspoons honey

2 ounces preserved ginger, drained, with 2–3 teaspoons syrup from the jar reserved

1 tablespoon chopped fresh mint

METHOD

1 Peel and seed the watermelon and finely chop the flesh. Put in a bowl. Working over the bowl to catch the juices, peel the grapefruit, removing and discarding most of the bitter white pith. Separate into segments, chop the flesh, and add to the watermelon.

2 Cut the chiles in half, remove and discard the seeds and membrane, and finely chop. Add to the fruit along with the honey. Stir well.

3 Finely chop the ginger and add to the bowl with the ginger syrup. Add the mint and stir well. Transfer the salsa to a serving bowl. Lightly cover and let stand in a cool place for 30 minutes to allow the flavors to develop. Stir again and serve.

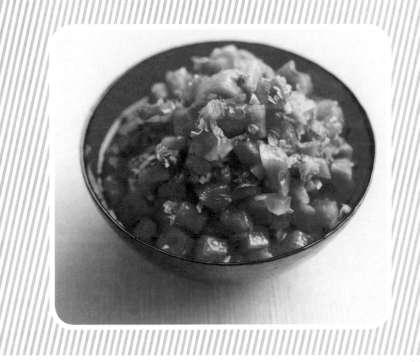

GRAPEFRUIT & AVOCADO SALAD

SERVES 2

1 pink grapefruit, peeled and cut into segments
2 avocados, sliced
½ red onion, finely sliced
2 cups mixed salad greens

DRESSING

4 dried dates, finely chopped
1 tablespoon olive oil
1 tablespoon walnut oil
1 tablespoon white wine vinegar

METHOD

1   To make the dressing, combine the finely chopped dates with the olive oil, walnut oil, and white wine vinegar in a small bowl, using a fork.

2   Place the grapefruit segments, avocado slices, and onion slices on a bed of fresh salad greens in a large salad bowl. Pour the dressing over the salad and toss, using two forks, to mix thoroughly. Serve immediately.

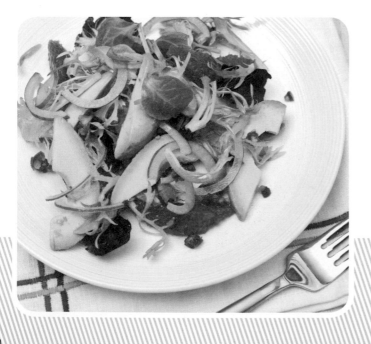

GRAPEFRUIT & CUCUMBER COOLER

SERVES 2

1 pound cucumbers, peeled
juice of 2 pink grapefruit

METHOD

1 Cut the cucumbers in half lengthwise and scoop out the seeds with a teaspoon. Coarsely chop the flesh.

2 Put the cucumber flesh into a food processor or blender with the grapefruit juice and process until thoroughly combined. Pour into a glass and serve immediately.

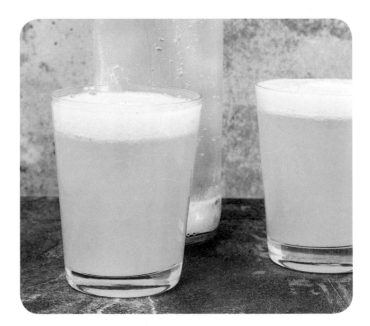

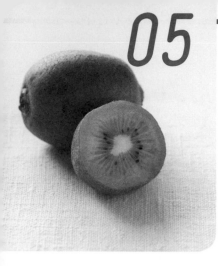

05

KIWIFRUIT

The kiwifruit has an unusual amount of omega-3 oils for a fruit. This, combined with its high vitamin C content, helps maintain healthy heart function.

MAJOR NUTRIENTS PER AVERAGE KIWIFRUIT

Calories	46
Total fat	0.39g
Protein	0.85g
Carbohydrate	11.06g
Fiber	2.26g
Vitamin C	69.9mg
Vitamin E	1.10mg
Potassium	235mg
Copper/Zeaxanthin	22.66mg
Calcium	25.64mcg
Zinc	0.10mcg
Omega-3 oils	31.75mg

Eating the edible seeds of fruits is extremely beneficial, and the seeds of the kiwi are particularly easy to swallow. As well as fiber and zinc, seeds contain all the nutrients and enzymes needed for a plant to grow, and when ingested they allow the body's cells to grow and regenerate. On average, kiwifruit seeds contain 62 percent alpha-linoleic acid, the omega-3 oil that helps protect the heart and decrease inflammation, both inside and outside the body. The kiwi is also a good source of copper, which is needed for collagen production and, therefore, healthy skin, nails, and muscles.

• Contains potassium, which helps regulate heart function.
• Contain more vitamin C than oranges, as well as vitamin E and rehydrating omega-3 oils for a skin-nourishing combination.
• Vitamin C works with copper to produce collagen, to keep skin renewed and firm.

Practical tips:
The kiwi can be eaten whole like an apple—eating the skin means you consume the vitamin C that lies just beneath it, and it vastly increases your intake of the fruit's insoluble fiber and antioxidant content. To test if a kiwi is ripe, press it—you should be able to depress the skin slightly, but the flesh beneath should be firm. Dried kiwi slices make healthy snacks, and can be bought in health-food stores.

GREEN GOODNESS

SERVES 2

1 pound cucumbers, peeled
4 kiwifruit, peeled
romaine lettuce leaves,
to garnish

METHOD

1 Cut the cucumber in half lengthwise and scoop out the seeds with a teaspoon. Coarsely chop the flesh.

2 Put the cucumber and kiwifruit into a food processor or blender and process until thoroughly combined. Pour into a glass, garnish with lettuce leaves, and serve immediately.

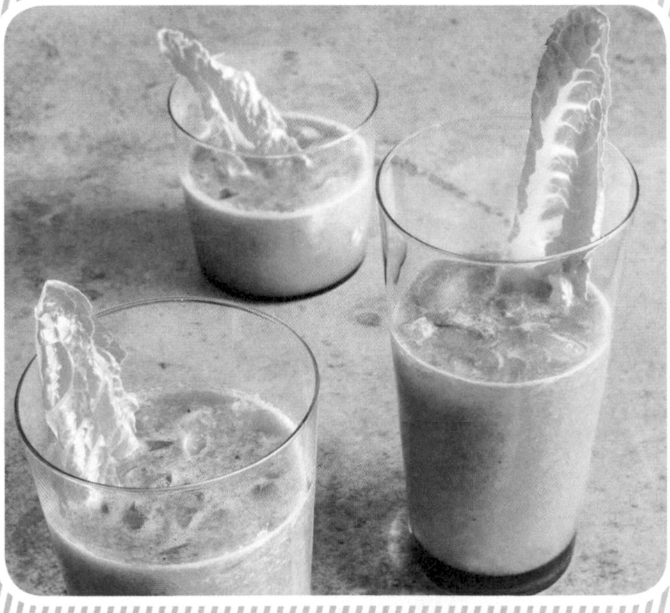

MIXED FRUIT KEBABS

SERVES 4

2 nectarines, halved
and pitted

2 kiwifruit

4 red plums

1 mango, peeled,
halved, and pitted

2 bananas, peeled
and thickly sliced

8 strawberries, hulled

1 tablespoon honey

3 tablespoons orange liqueur

METHOD

1 Cut the nectarine halves into wedges and place in a large, shallow dish. Peel and quarter the kiwis. Cut the plums in half and remove the pits. Cut the mango flesh into chunks and add to the dish with the kiwis, plums, bananas, and strawberries.

2 Mix the honey and liqueur together in a measuring cup until blended. Pour the mixture over the fruit and toss to coat. Cover with plastic wrap and let marinate in the refrigerator for 1 hour.

3 Preheat the broiler to high. Drain the fruit, reserving the marinade. Thread the fruit onto several metal or presoaked wooden skewers and cook under the preheated broiler, turning and brushing frequently with the reserved marinade, for 5–7 minutes. Serve immediately.

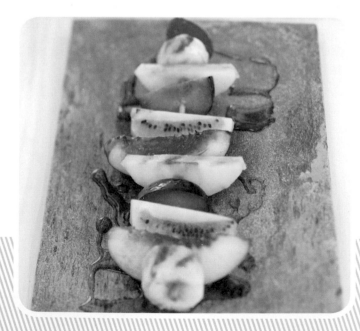

KIWI SORBET

SERVES 6

1 pound 9 ounces kiwifruit
4 tablespoons orange juice
¾ cup granulated sugar
strip of thinly pared
lemon rind

METHOD

1 Peel all of the kiwis and roughly chop the flesh. Put them into a food processor with the orange juice and process until pureed.

2 Put the sugar and lemon rind in a heavy-based saucepan and pour in ¾ cup water. Bring to a boil, stirring until the sugar has dissolved, then remove the pan from the heat and set aside.

3 Remove and discard the lemon rind from the sugar syrup. Stir in the kiwi fruit puree and mix well. Pour the mixture into a freezer-proof container, cover, and place in the freezer for 1 hour until ice crystals have formed around the edges. Scoop the sorbet into the blender and process until smooth. Return to the container and replace in the freezer for 1 hour.

4 Process the sorbet in the blender again, then return to the freezer. Repeat this process once more, then freeze until firm. Transfer the container to the refrigerator 10 minutes before serving to allow the sorbet to soften slightly.

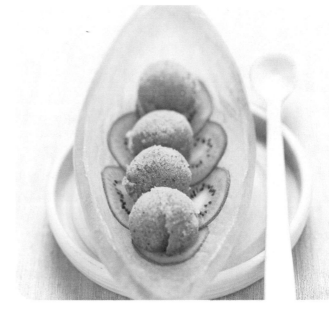

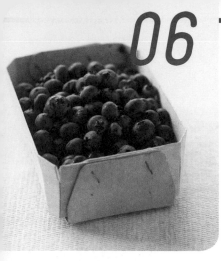

06

BLUEBERRIES

These deep-purple berries are the richest of all fruits in antioxidant compounds, which could help protect the body from various diseases.

MAJOR NUTRIENTS PER ⅓ CUP/1¾ OUNCES BLUEBERRIES

Calories	29
Total fat	Trace
Protein	0.4g
Carbohydrate	7.2g
Fiber	1.2g
Vitamin C	5mg
Vitamin E	2.4mg
Folate	34mcg
Potassium	39mg
Lutein/Zeaxanthin	40mcg

The blueberry was one of the first fruits to be named a superfood, and it's thought that just a handful of berries a day could offer protection from some diseases. The compound pterostilbene, which is found in the fruit, could be as effective as commercial medicines in lowering cholesterol, and may also help prevent diabetes and some cancers. Blueberries are also a good source of anthocyanins, which can help to prevent heart disease and memory loss. They are high in vitamin C and fiber and also appear to help urinary tract infections.

- Contain a cholesterol-lowering compound.
- Can help prevent coronary heart disease, diabetes, and some cancers.
- Could help to treat urinary tract infections.
- Lutein and zeaxanthin helps keep eyes healthy.

Practical tips:
Blueberries are sweet and ideally should be eaten raw, which helps to preserve their vitamin C content. Store in a nonmetallic container, because contact with metal can discolor them. Blueberries are a valuable kitchen staple and can boost the nutrient content of muffins, cakes, crisps, pies, and fruit salads. The berries freeze well and lose few of their nutrients in the process.

TURKEY & BLUEBERRY SALAD

SERVES 4

10½ ounces cold roast turkey

10½ ounces celery sticks, sliced

1½ cups blueberries

2½ ounces walnuts, roughly chopped

DRESSING

3½ ounces blue cheese, such as Roquefort or Gorgonzola

3½ ounces crème fraîche

2 tablespoons lemon juice

salt and pepper, to taste

METHOD

1 Cut the turkey into bite-size pieces and place in a large bowl with the celery, blueberries, and half the walnuts. Toss together to mix evenly.

2 To make the dressing, mash the blue cheese with a fork, then stir in the crème fraîche and lemon juice. Season with salt and pepper.

3 Stir the dressing into the salad, mixing evenly. Spoon into individual serving bowls, scatter the remaining walnuts over the top and serve immediately.

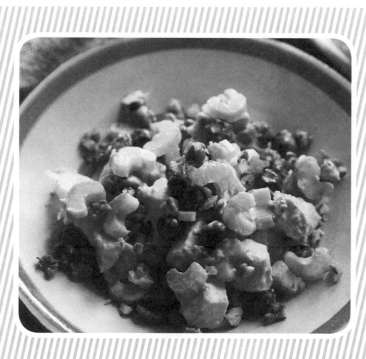

BLUEBERRY CORNMEAL PANCAKES

SERVES 2

1 cup all-purpose flour
1½ teaspoons baking powder
½ cup cornmeal
2 tablespoons superfine sugar
pinch of salt
1¼ cups buttermilk
2 large eggs
½ stick butter, melted
4 cups blueberries
confectioners' sugar and
maple syrup, to serve

METHOD

1 Mix together the flour, baking powder, cornmeal, sugar, and salt in a large bowl. In a second bowl, whisk the buttermilk, eggs, and half the melted butter until smooth. Stir the buttermilk mixture into the flour mixture and beat to form a batter. Fold in the blueberries lightly, taking care not to crush them.

2 Place a non-stick skillet over medium-high heat and brush with some of the remaining melted butter. Drop 2–3 tablespoons of the mixture into the skillet and cook for 1–2 minutes, or until bubbles appear on the surface. Turn the pancake over and cook for a further minute until golden. Keep warm, while making the remaining pancakes, brushing the skillet with melted butter between batches.

3 Stack three to four pancakes on each plate and dust with confectioners' sugar. Drizzle with maple syrup and serve. Any leftover pancakes can be placed in the refrigerator and served later, spread with butter.

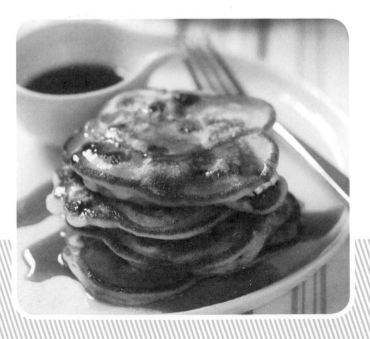

BLUEBERRY & OATMEAL MUFFINS

MAKES 9

1 cup orange juice
⅔ cup rolled oats
½ cup granulated sugar
1⅔ cups all-purpose flour, sifted
½ teaspoon xanthan gum
1½ teaspoons baking powder
½ teaspoon baking soda
½ teaspoon cinnamon
¼ teaspoon allspice
½ cup vegetable oil
1 egg, beaten
1 teaspoon glycerin
1¼ cups blueberries
raw brown sugar, to sprinkle

METHOD

1 Preheat the oven to 350°F. Line a deep 9-cup muffin pan with muffin cups.

2 Add the orange juice to the rolled oats and mix well in a bowl.

3 In a separate bowl, mix together the sugar, flour, xanthan gum, baking powder, baking soda, and spices. Add the oil, egg, and glycerin to the dry mixture and mix well. Then add the oat mixture and blueberries and fold these in gently.

4 Divide the batter among the muffin cups and sprinkle each muffin with raw sugar.

5 Bake the muffins in the preheated oven for 20–25 minutes, or until a toothpick inserted in a muffin comes out clean. Remove from the oven and cool on a wire rack.

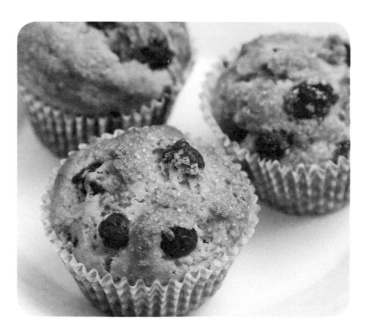

07

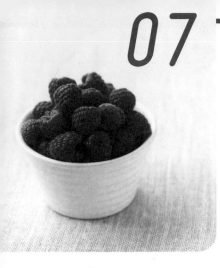

RASPBERRIES

Packed with vitamin C, fiber, and antioxidants to protect the heart, raspberries are one of the most nutritious fruits.

Raspberries are a surprisingly nutritious fruit, best eaten raw, because cooking or processing destroys some of the antioxidants, especially anthocyanins. Anthocyanins are naturally occurring red and purple pigments that have been shown to help prevent both heart disease and certain cancers, and may also help to prevent varicose veins. Raspberries also contain high levels of ellagic acid, a compound with anticancer properties. In addition, they are high in fiber and contain good amounts of iron, which the body absorbs well because of the accompanying high levels of vitamin C.

- High antioxidant content.
- May help to prevent varicose veins.
- One portion contains approximately half a day's recommended intake of vitamin C.
- High fiber content helps lower bad cholesterol.

Practical tips:
Raspberries do not stay fresh for long, so they should be picked only when ripe and should be consumed relatively quickly. They do, however, freeze well, but they should be packed in single layers in plastic containers, not in plastic bags. Never wash raspberries before storing unless absolutely necessary—their structure is easily destroyed. The healthy soluble fiber in raspberries is pectin, which means they make excellent easy-to-set preserves.

MAJOR NUTRIENTS PER ¾ CUP/3½ OUNCES RASPBERRIES

Calories	52
Total fat	0.6g
Protein	1.2g
Carbohydrate	12g
Fiber	6.5g
Vitamin C	26mg
Vitamin B3	0.8mg
Vitamin E	0.6mg
Folate	21mg
Potassium	151mg
Calcium	25mg
Iron	0.7mg
Zinc	0.4mg

DID YOU KNOW?

Raspberries consist of smaller fruits called drupelets, which are clustered around a stalk core in the center. Each drupelet contains a seed, which is why raspberries are so high in fiber.

RASPBERRY & PEAR REFRESHER

SERVES 2

2 large, ripe Bartlett pears
1 cup frozen raspberries
1 cup ice-cold water
honey, to taste

METHOD

1 Peel and quarter the pears, removing the cores. Place the pears in a food processor or blender with the raspberries and water and process until smooth.

2 Taste and sweeten with honey to taste. Pour into chilled glasses and serve.

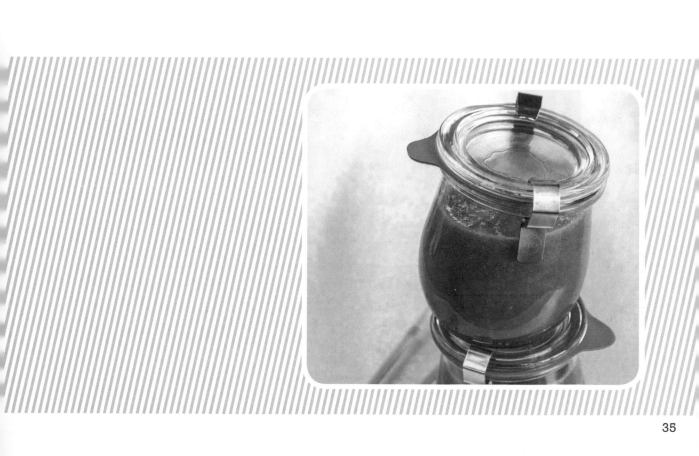

RASPBERRY & LEMON CUPCAKES

MAKES 12

1 stick butter, softened

¾ cup granulated sugar

2 large eggs, lightly beaten

1 cup all-purpose flour

1½ teaspoons baking powder

finely grated rind of 1 lemon

1 tablespoon lemon curd

¾ cup fresh raspberries

TOPPING

2 tablespoons butter

1 tablespoon soft light brown sugar

1 tablespoon almond meal (ground almonds)

1 tablespoon all-purpose flour

METHOD

1 Preheat the oven to 400°F. Put 12 paper muffin cups into a muffin pan or put 12 double-layer muffin cups onto baking sheets.

2 To make the topping, put the butter in a saucepan and heat gently until melted. Pour into a bowl and add the sugar, ground almonds and flour and stir together until combined.

3 To make the cupcakes, put the butter and sugar in a large bowl and beat together until light and fluffy, then gradually add the eggs. Sift together the flour and baking powder and fold into the mixture. Fold in the lemon rind, lemon curd and raspberries. Spoon the mixture into the paper cases. Add the topping to cover the top of each cupcake and press down gently.

4 Bake in the preheated oven for 15–20 minutes, or until golden brown and firm to the touch. Leave the cupcakes to cool for 10 minutes, then transfer to a wire rack to cool completely.

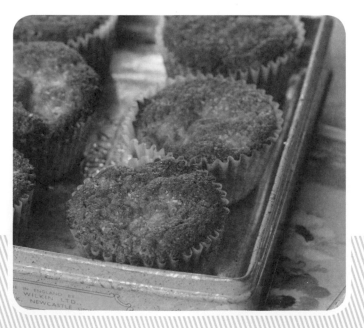

RASPBERRY OAT SLICES

MAKES 16

1⅔ cups all-purpose flour

1 teaspoon baking powder

½ cup superfine sugar

½ cup lightly packed light brown sugar

1 cup butter

1 teaspoon almond extract

1¾ cups rolled oats

⅔ cup raspberry conserve

½ cup slivered almonds

METHOD

1   Preheat the oven to 375°F Line a 12 x 8-inch rectangular baking pan. Sift the flour and baking powder into a large bowl, add the sugars, and mix well. Add the butter and rub it in with your fingertips until the mixture resembles bread crumbs. Stir in the almond extract and oats, then press three-quarters of the mixture into the bottom of the pan. Bake in the preheated oven for 10 minutes.

2   Spread the conserve over the cooked base and sprinkle it with half of the almonds.

3   Put the remaining flour mixture and the remaining almonds in a bowl and mix together, then sprinkle evenly over the top and press down gently. Bake for an additional 20–25 minutes, or until golden brown. Let cool in the pan, then cut into slices to serve.

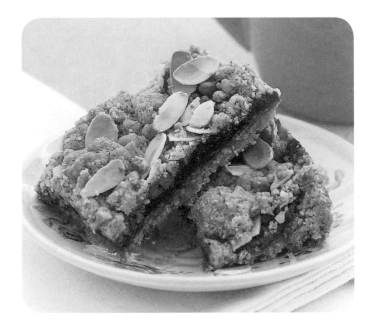

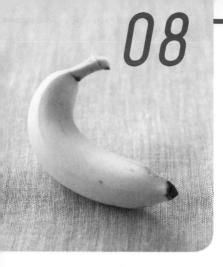

08

BANANAS

The banana is the ultimate sports snack because it provides quick, quality fuel for the body. It is perfect for replenishing and repairing flagging cells.

Bananas are high in sugar, but they shouldn't be underestimated for their health-giving properties. A ripe banana contains a high amount of fiber, including the prebiotic inulin, which feeds our beneficial (probiotic) digestive bacteria, the first line of defense for the immune system. Keeping your digestive bacteria healthy can help prevent inflammatory conditions such as eczema, asthma, and arthritis, and it supports the digestion and absorption of nutrients needed to maintain optimal health.

- Potassium and vitamin C help transport oxygen around the body to renew and revitalize the skin.
- Contain high levels of potassium, vitamin C, and vitamin B6, which are all important for heart health.
- Athletes draw on the rich nutritional mixture in bananas to support performance, recovery, and muscle response.
- Proven to help kidney function and eliminate fluid retention, reducing puffiness for a more youthful appearance.

Practical tips:
The fruit of choice for many people with a sweet tooth, bananas are best eaten when the skin is a solid yellow color, with no bruises. Avoid overripe, brown bananas because, by this stage, the sugars will have broken down and the fruit becomes soft and sweet. Bananas may not be suitable for people with phlegm and nasal congestion, because they can make these conditions worse.

MAJOR NUTRIENTS PER AVERAGE BANANA

Calories	105
Total fat	0.39g
Protein	1.29g
Carbohydrate	26.95g
Fiber	3.1g
Vitamin B6	0.43mg
Vitamin C	10.3mg
Potassium	422mg

DID YOU KNOW?

The name "banana" comes from the Arabic banan, which means "finger"—they grow in clusters of up to 20 fruit called a "hand."

BANANA & STRAWBERRY SMOOTHIE

SERVES 2

1 banana, sliced

4 ounces strawberries, hulled

⅔ cup plain yogurt with live cultures

METHOD

1   Put the banana, strawberries, and yogurt into a food processor or blender and process for a few seconds until smooth. Pour into glasses and serve immediately.

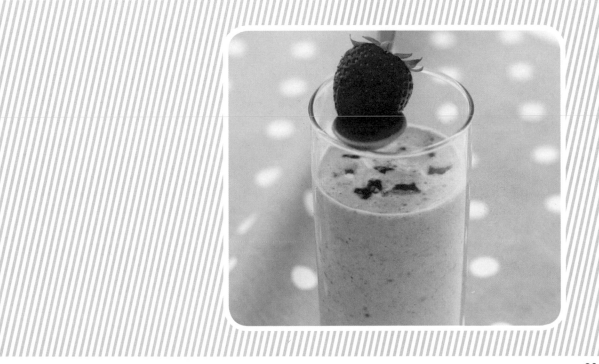

BANANA STREUSEL BARS

MAKES 10

1¾ sticks butter, plus extra for greasing

½ cup firmly packed dark brown sugar

1⅔ cups rolled oats

½ cup chopped pecans

½ teaspoon ground cinnamon

½ cup granulated sugar

2 eggs, lightly beaten

⅔ cup mashed, peeled ripe banana

1⅔ cups all-purpose flour

2½ teaspoons baking powder

METHOD

1 Preheat the oven to 350°F. Grease a 7-inch square cake pan and line with nonstick parchment paper. Place ¾ stick of the butter and the brown sugar in a saucepan over low heat and stir until melted and smooth. Remove from the heat. Stir in the oats, nuts, and cinnamon. Set aside.

2 Beat together the remaining 1 stick of butter and the granulated sugar until creamy, and gradually add the eggs, beating well after each addition. Fold in the banana, flour, and baking powder with a large metal spoon.

3 Spread half the cake batter over the bottom of the prepared pan. Sprinkle half the oat mixture over the top, then repeat the layers once. Bake in the preheated oven for 50–60 minutes, until risen and the center is firm to the touch. Let cool in the pan for about 1 hour, then turn out and cut into ten bars.

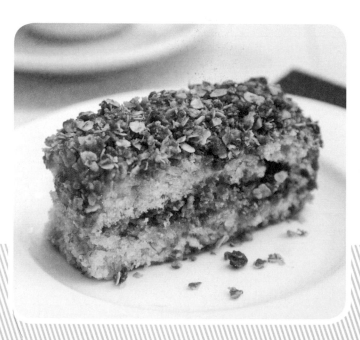

HONEY BANANA MUFFINS

MAKES 12

2¼ cups all-purpose flour

3 teaspoons baking powder

½ teaspoon baking soda

1 teaspoon ground cinnamon

pinch of salt

½ cup granulated sugar

¾ stick butter, melted

½ cup milk

2 tablespoons honey,
plus extra for brushing

1 teaspoon vanilla extract

2 large eggs

2 ripe bananas, mashed

dried banana chips,
to decorate

METHOD

1   Preheat the oven to 350°F. Line a muffin pan with muffin cups. Sift the flour, baking powder, baking soda, cinnamon, and salt into a large bowl. Add the sugar and stir to combine.

2   In a second bowl, beat the melted butter, milk, honey, vanilla extract, eggs, and mashed banana together. Add to the flour mixture and stir lightly and thoroughly until just combined.

3   Divide the mixture evenly among the paper cases. Bake in the preheated oven for 20–25 minutes, or until well risen. Brush the top of each muffin with honey and top with a banana chip. Leave to cool in the pan for 15 minutes before transferring to a wire rack. Serve two muffins each for breakfast, either warm or at room temperature.

4   The remaining muffins will freeze for up to 2 months. When ready to use, defrost thoroughly and warm through in the oven.

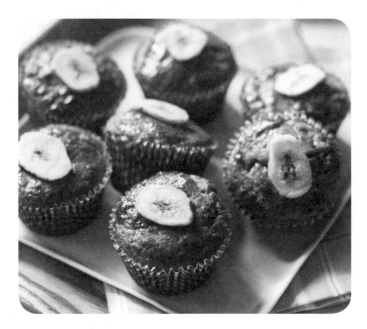

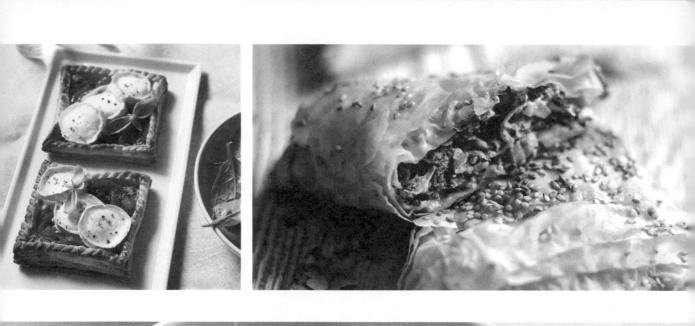

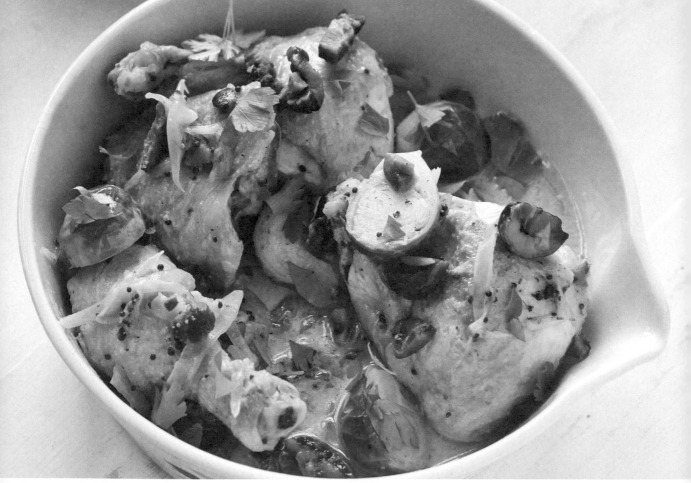

VEGETABLES

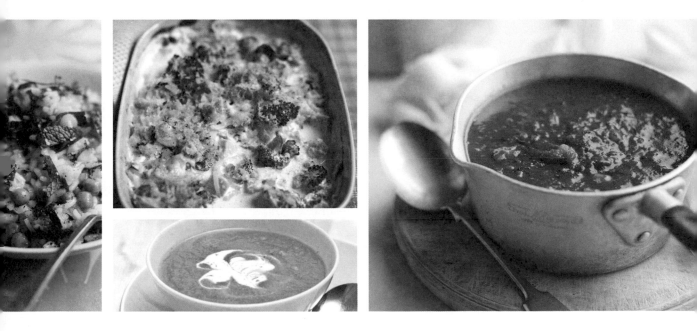

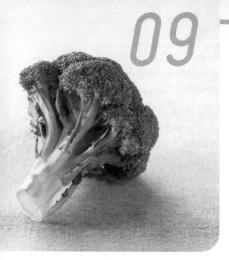

09

BROCCOLI

Of all the vegetables in the brassica (cabbage) family, broccoli, with its high levels of selenium, has shown the highest levels of protection against prostate cancer.

**MAJOR NUTRIENTS PER
1 CUP/ 3½ OUNCES
CHOPPED BROCCOLI**

Calories	34
Total fat	0.4g
Protein	2.8g
Carbohydrate	6.6g
Fiber	2.6g
Vitamin C	89mg
Selenium	2.5mcg
Beta-carotene	361mcg
Calcium	47mg
Lutein/Zeaxanthin	1,403mcg

Broccoli comes in several varieties, but the darker the color, the more beneficial nutrients the vegetable contains. It contains sulforaphane and indoles, which have been shown to help prevent cancer, particularly in the breast and colon. Broccoli is also high in flavonoids, which have been specifically linked to a significant reduction in the risk of ovarian cancer. The chemicals in broccoli are also thought to protect against stomach ulcers. They act as a detoxifier, helping to lower bad blood cholesterol, boost the immune system, and protect against cataracts.

- Rich in a variety of nutrients that protect against types of cancer.
- Lutein and zeaxanthin help prevent macular degeneration.
- Helps eradicate the *H. pylori* bacteria, encouraging a healthy digestive tract.
- High calcium content helps build and protect bones.
- Excellent source of the antioxidants vitamin C and selenium.

Practical tips:
Look for broccoli heads that are rich in color and avoid any with pale, yellow, or brown patches on the florets. You can eat the leaves and stems of broccoli, which are also nutritionally beneficial. Frozen broccoli contains all the nutrients of fresh broccoli, and offers a more convenient storage method. Cook by lightly steaming or stir-frying.

BROCCOLI & PEANUT STIR-FRY

SERVES 4

3 tablespoons vegetable oil or peanut oil

1 lemongrass stalk, coarsely chopped

2 fresh red chiles, seeded and chopped

1-inch piece fresh ginger, peeled and grated

3 kaffir lime leaves, coarsely torn

3 tablespoons Thai green curry paste

1 onion, chopped

1 red bell pepper, seeded and chopped

5 cups broccoli florets

1 cup trimmed green beans

⅓ cup toasted unsalted peanuts

METHOD

1 Put 2 tablespoons of the oil, the lemongrass, chiles, ginger, lime leaves, and curry paste in a food processor or blender and process until a paste forms.

2 Heat a wok or skillet over high heat. Add the remaining oil and heat for 30 seconds. Add the spice paste, onion, and red bell pepper and stir-fry for 2–3 minutes, until the vegetables start to soften.

3 Add the broccoli and beans, cover, and cook over low heat for 4–5 minutes, until tender.

4 Add the peanuts to the wok, toss to mix, and serve.

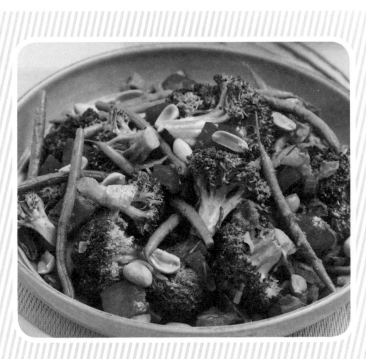

BROCCOLI SOUP

SERVES 6

½ head of broccoli
1 leek, sliced
1 celery stalk, sliced
1 clove garlic, crushed
3 Yukon gold, red-skinnned, or white round potatoes, diced
4 cups vegetable stock
1 bay leaf
pepper, to taste
toasted croutons, to serve

METHOD

1   Cut the broccoli into florets and set aside. Cut the thicker broccoli stems into ½-inch dice and put into a large saucepan with the leek, celery, garlic, potato, stock, and bay leaf. Bring to a boil, then reduce the heat, cover, and simmer for 15 minutes.

2   Add the broccoli florets to the soup and return to a boil. Reduce the heat, cover, and simmer for an additional 3–5 minutes, or until the potato and broccoli stems are tender.

3   Remove from the heat and let the soup cool slightly. Remove and discard the bay leaf. Transfer to a food processor or blender, in batches if necessary, and process until smooth.

4   Return the soup to the saucepan and heat through thoroughly. Season with pepper. Ladle the soup into warm bowls and serve immediately, sprinkled with toasted croutons.

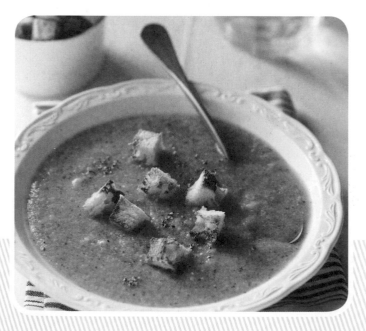

CHICKEN & BROCCOLI CASSEROLE

SERVES 4

1 head of broccoli, cut into florets

3 tablespoons butter

1 onion, thinly sliced

2½ cups bite-size cooked chicken chunks

½ cup crème fraîche or sour cream

1 cup chicken stock

½ cup fresh white bread crumbs

½ cup shredded Swiss cheese

salt and pepper, to taste

METHOD

1 Preheat the oven to 400°F. Bring a saucepan of lightly salted water to a boil, add the broccoli, and cook for 5 minutes, until tender. Drain well.

2 Meanwhile, melt 2 tablespoons of the butter in a skillet, add the onion, and sauté over medium heat, stirring, for 3–4 minutes, until soft.

3 Layer the broccoli, onion, and chicken in a 1½-quart casserole dish and season well with salt and pepper. Pour the crème fraîche and stock over the chicken and vegetables.

4 Melt the remaining butter in a small saucepan and stir in the bread crumbs. Mix with the cheese and sprinkle the mixture over the dish.

5 Place the dish on a baking sheet in the preheated oven and bake for 20–25 minutes, until golden brown and bubbling. Serve hot.

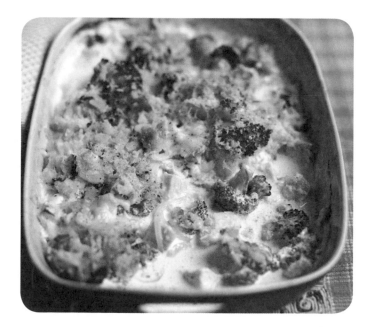

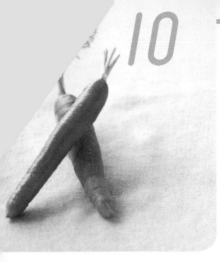

10

CARROTS

The richest in carotenes of all plant foods, carrots offer protection from cancers and cardiovascular disease, and they help keep eyes and lungs healthy.

MAJOR NUTRIENTS PER AVERAGE CARROT

Calories	41
Total fat	Trace
Protein	0.9g
Carbohydrate	9.6g
Fiber	2.8g
Vitamin C	6mg
Vitamin E	0.7mg
Beta-carotene	8,285mcg
Calcium	33mg
Potassium	320mg
Lutein/Zeaxanthin	256mcg

Carrots are one of the most nutritious root vegetables. They are an excellent source of antioxidant compounds and the richest vegetable source of carotenes, which give them their bright-orange color. These compounds help protect against cardiovascular disease and cancer. Carotenes may reduce the risk of heart disease by about 45 percent, promote good vision, and help maintain healthy lungs. They are also rich in fiber, antioxidant vitamins C and E, calcium, and potassium. There is ongoing research into the effect of falcarinol, a chemical in carrots, in suppressing tumors.

- High carotene content protects against high blood cholesterol and heart disease.
- May offer protection against some cancers and emphysema.
- Women who eat at least five carrots a week are nearly two-thirds less likely to have a stroke than those who don't.
- Help protect sight and night vision.
- Contain a good range of vitamins, minerals, and fiber.

Practical tips:
The darker orange the carrot, the more carotenes it will contain. Remove any green on the stem end of the carrot before cooking, because it can be mildly toxic. The nutrients in carrots are more available to the body when a carrot is cooked, compared with when eaten raw, and adding a little vegetable oil during cooking helps the carotenes to be absorbed.

DID YOU KNOW?

A very high intake of carrots can cause the skin to appear orange—called carotenemia, it is a harmless condition.

VICHY CARROTS

SERVES 4–6

2 tablespoons unsalted butter

6 carrots (about 1 pound), cut into ¼-inch slices

1 tablespoon sugar

bottle of Vichy mineral water

salt and pepper

2 tablespoons chopped fresh flat-leaf parsley

METHOD

1 Melt the butter in a large, heavy saucepan over medium–high heat. Stir in the carrots, then stir in the sugar and season with salt and pepper.

2 Pour over enough Vichy water to cover the carrots by 2 inches and bring to a boil. Reduce the heat to medium and let the carrots simmer, uncovered, stirring occasionally, until they are tender, all the liquid has been absorbed, and they are coated in a thin glaze.

3 Adjust the seasoning, if necessary, transfer to a serving dish, and stir in the parsley. Serve immediately.

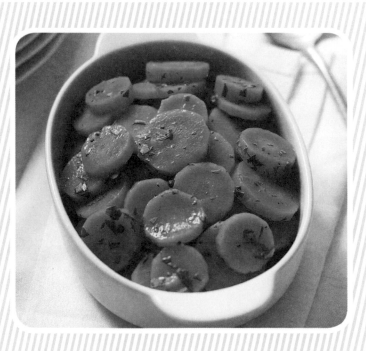

CARROT CAKE WITH CREAM CHEESE FROSTING

SERVES 12

2½ cups finely grated carrots
2 cups all-purpose flour
1½ cups sugar
½ cup firmly packed brown sugar
2 teaspoons baking soda
1 teaspoon baking powder
2 teaspoons ground cinnamon
4 eggs, beaten
1⅓ cups vegetable oil, plus extra for greasing
1⅓ teaspoons vanilla extract

FROSTING

1 cup cream cheese
½ cup unsalted butter
3 cups confectioners' sugar
2 teaspoons vanilla extract
1 cup chopped pecans

METHOD

1 Preheat the oven to 350°F. Grease 3 x 9-inch round cake pans.

2 In a large mixing bowl combine the grated carrots, flour, sugar, brown sugar, soda, baking powder, and cinnamon. Stir well to combine. In a separate bowl combine the eggs, oil, and vanilla

3 Add the wet ingredients to the dry ingredients, mixing until smooth. Pour the batter into the prepared cake pans. Bake in the preheated oven for 30 minutes, or until a toothpick inserted in the center comes out clean. Let the cakes cool in the pans for 5 minutes, then remove them from the pans and let cool completely on wire racks.

4 To make the cream cheese frosting, combine the cream cheese and butter, beating until smooth. Add the sugar and vanilla and beat until light and fluffy. Stir in the pecans and then spread between the layers of the cake, and on top.

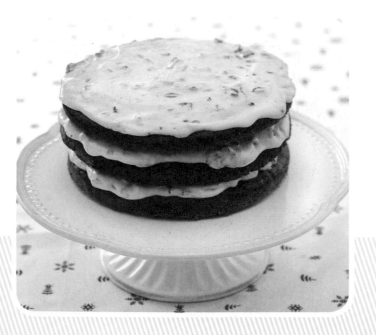

CARROT & CUMIN SOUP

SERVES 2

1 carrot, finely chopped

1 garlic clove, chopped

1 shallot, finely chopped

1 ripe tomato, skinned
and chopped

½ teaspoon ground cumin

1 cup vegetable stock

1 bouquet garni (sprigs of
parsley, thyme, and a bay
leaf tied together)

pepper, to taste

pinch of cumin and
1 tablespoon reduced-fat
crème fraîche or Greek
yogurt (optional), to garnish

METHOD

1   Put the carrot, garlic, shallot, tomato, cumin, stock, and bouquet
    garni in a lidded saucepan.

2   Bring to a simmering point over high heat, then reduce the heat
    and simmer for 30 minutes, or until the vegetables are tender.
    Let cool slightly and remove the bouquet garni.

3   Pour the soup into a food processor or blender and puree
    until smooth.

4   Return to the saucepan and reheat gently. Season with pepper.
    Remove from the heat and ladle into warm mugs or bowls.
    Garnish with cumin and a swirl of crème fraîche or Greek
    yogurt, if using, and serve.

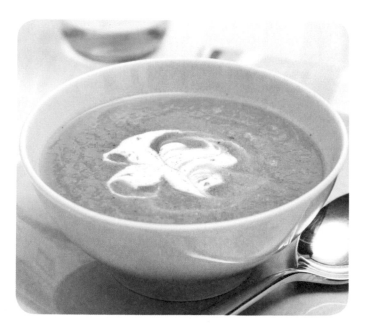

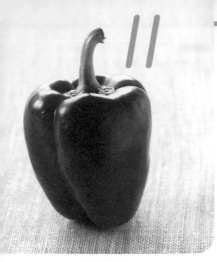

RED BELL PEPPERS

All members of the capsicum family, which includes chiles and paprika, have fantastic youth-preserving benefits, and are especially good for the heart and skin.

MAJOR NUTRIENTS PER AVERAGE RED BELL PEPPER

Calories	37
Total fat	0.36g
Protein	1.18g
Carbohydrate	7.18g
Fiber	2.5g
Vitamin A	6,681 IU
Vitamin C	222mg
Vitamin B6	0.35mg
Folate	25.7mcg

The color of red bell peppers comes from the antioxidant carotenoid lycopene, just one of the nutrients that distinguishes them from green bell peppers. They also contain twice the amount of vitamin C and around nine times the carotene as their green counterparts. An important part of the youth-preserving Mediterranean diet, red bell peppers contribute to heart health, because their high levels of antioxidants keep the arteries in good condition. The vitamin B6 and folate present also help to reduce levels of homocysteine, a substance we produce naturally but that is linked to heart disease and dementia if levels become high.

- Rich source of a range of vitamins, minerals, and plant chemicals.
- Contain vitamin A stops the damage to skin from UV light that can be seen as wrinkles and age spots.
- Contain vitamin C and vitamin B6, which are needed to make stomach acid: vital for killing off harmful bacteria.
- Contain folate, needed for cell growth and skin renewal.

Practical tip:
A bell pepper should feel weighty and have a healthy green stem. The skin should be smooth, firm, and wrinkle-free. Avoid bell peppers with indents or black spots. Store, unwashed, in a plastic bag in the refrigerator for up to a week. Fat-soluble carotenoids need oil to carry them into the body, so eating red bell peppers with olive oil will double their health value and optimize their absorption by the body.

RED BELL PEPPER DIP

SERVES 6

2 red bell peppers, halved and seeded

2 garlic cloves

1 tablespoon olive oil

1 tablespoon lemon juice

½ cup fresh white bread crumbs

salt and pepper, to taste

METHOD

1   Place the bell pepper halves and garlic in a pan and add just enough water to cover. Bring to a boil, then reduce the heat, cover, and simmer gently for 10–15 minutes until soft and tender. Drain and set aside to cool.

2   Coarsely chop the bell pepper halves and garlic and place in a food processor with the olive oil and lemon juice. Process to a smooth paste.

3   Add the bread crumbs and process briefly until just combined. Season with salt and pepper to taste. Transfer to a serving bowl, cover with plastic wrap, and chill in the refrigerator until required.

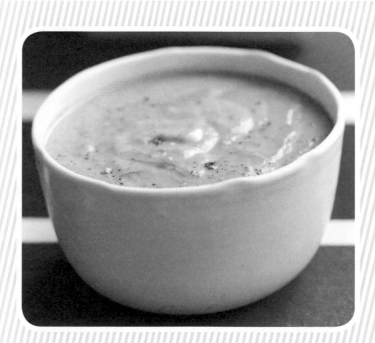

RED BELL PEPPER SMOOTHIE

SERVES 2

1 cup carrot juice
1 cup tomato juice
2 large red bell peppers,
seeded and coarsely
chopped
1 tablespoon lemon juice
pepper
lemon slices, to garnish

METHOD

1   Pour the carrot juice and tomato juice into a food processor or blender and process gently until combined.

2   Add the red bell peppers and lemon juice. Season with plenty of pepper and process until smooth. Pour the mixture into glasses, garnish with lemon slices, and serve.

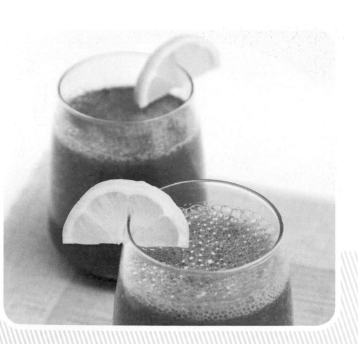

GOAT'S CHEESE & RED BELL PEPPER TARTS

MAKES 2

7 ounces store-bought puff pastry

flour, to dust

1 large egg, beaten

2 red peppers

4 tablespoons ready-made pesto

4 ounces goat's cheese, sliced

fresh basil sprigs, to garnish

METHOD

1　Preheat the oven to 400°F. Roll out the pastry on a lightly floured surface.

2　Cut the pastry into two pieces and transfer to a baking sheet. With the tip of a sharp knife, score a line about ½ inch inside the edge all the way around. Make diagonal scores on the outside rim of the pastry and brush this with beaten egg. Bake in the preheated oven for 10 minutes, or until risen and golden.

3　Meanwhile, char the peppers over a gas flame or under a preheated broiler until blackened all over. Wrap the peppers in aluminum foil and leave to cool a little. Scrape off the charred skin, rinse under cold water and remove the stalk and seeds. Thinly slice the peppers.

4　Cut along the inner line of the pastry cases to loosen the centre part and push down gently. Spread 2 tablespoons of pesto in the centre part of each tart then arrange the sliced peppers on top. Lay slices of goat's cheese on each one and return to the oven for 5 minutes, or until the goat's cheese has melted. Serve the tarts immediately, garnished with basil sprigs.

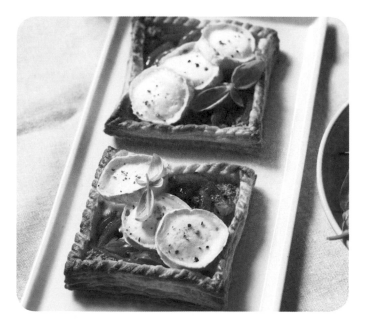

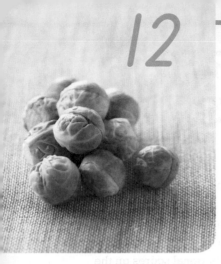

12

BRUSSELS SPROUTS

Brussels sprouts are packed with immune-boosting nutrients, and they should be consumed regularly to enjoy their potential health benefits.

MAJOR NUTRIENTS PER 5 BRUSSELS SPROUTS

Calories	43
Total fat	0.3g
Protein	3.4g
Carbohydrate	9g
Fiber	3.8g
Vitamin C	85mg
Folate	61mcg
Magnesium	23mg
Calcium	42mg
Selenium	1.6mcg
Zinc	0.4mg
Beta-carotene	450mcg
Lutein/Zeaxanthin	1,590mcg

Brussels sprouts are an important winter vegetable, providing high levels of vitamin C and many other immune-boosting nutrients. They are rich in the sulforaphane compound, which is a detoxifier and has been shown to help the body clear itself of potential carcinogens. Brussels sprouts have been shown to help prevent DNA damage when eaten regularly and may help minimize the spread of breast cancer. They even contain small amounts of beneficial omega-3 fats, zinc, and selenium, a mineral many adults do not eat in the recommended daily amount. People who eat large quantities of brussels sprouts and other brassicas (cabbage family vegetables) are thought to have a much lower risk of prostate, colorectal, and lung cancers.

• Rich in indoles and other compounds to protect against cancer, sprouts may also reduce the spread of cancer.
• Extremely rich in immune-boosting vitamin C.
• Indole content can also help lower bad blood cholesterol.
• Very high in fiber, which is good for digestive health.

Practical tips:
Select bright-green sprouts with tight heads and no sign of yellow leaves. Lightly steaming or quickly boiling brussels sprouts is the best way to cook them and preserve their nutrients. Don't overcook because much of the vitamin C content will be destroyed. Overcooking also alters their flavor and gives them an unwelcome odor.

PECAN-GLAZED BRUSSELS SPROUTS

SERVES 6

1½ pounds fresh brussels sprouts

½ cup water

¼ cup unsalted butter or margarine

⅓ cup firmly packed brown sugar

3 tablespoons soy sauce

¼ teaspoon salt

½ cup finely chopped pecans, toasted

METHOD

1 Wash the brussels sprouts thoroughly, and remove any discolored leaves. Cut off the stem ends, and slash the bottom of each sprout with a shallow "X." Bring ½ cup water to a boil in a large saucepan; add the brussels sprouts. Cover, reduce the heat, and simmer for 8 to 10 minutes, or until sprouts are tender; drain and set aside.

2 Melt the butter in a medium skillet; stir in the brown sugar, soy sauce, and salt. Bring the butter mixture to a boil, stirring constantly. Add pecans; reduce the heat, and simmer, uncovered, for 5 minutes, stirring occasionally. Add the brussels sprouts; cook over medium heat for 5 minutes; stir well before serving.

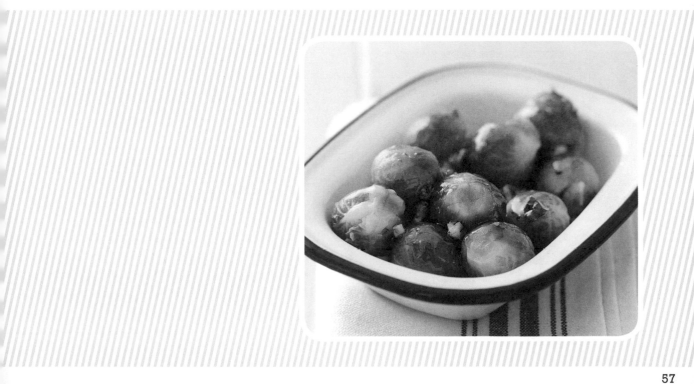

BRAISED CHICKEN WITH BRUSSELS SPROUTS

SERVES 4

2 tablespoons olive oil

1 whole chicken (about
3 pounds) cut into 8 pieces

4 ounces smoked bacon

2 onions, finely sliced

2 garlic cloves, finely sliced

3½ ounces cooked and
peeled chestnuts, halved

1 cup hard cider

1 cup chicken stock

9 ounces brussels sprouts,
trimmed and halved

1 tablespoon whole-grain
mustard

2 tablespoons heavy cream

small handful parsley,
leaves chopped

METHOD

1   Heat half of the oil in a large flameproof casserole over medium-high heat, add the chicken in batches, and brown all over. Remove and set to one side.

2   Add the bacon to the casserole and fry until starting to crisp. Remove with a slotted spoon and set aside with the chicken. Add the onion to the casserole and fry gently in the bacon fat until softened. Stir in the garlic and cook for a further 2–3 minutes.

3   Return the chicken and bacon to the casserole and add the chestnuts. Pour in the cider and allow it to bubble for 2–3 minutes. Pour in the stock, cover, and cook over medium heat for 30 minutes, uncovering for the final 5 minutes, until the chicken is cooked through.

4   Add the sprouts, pushing them into the cooking liquid, re-cover and bubble for a final 5 minutes. Stir in the mustard and cream and finish with a sprinkling of chopped parsley.

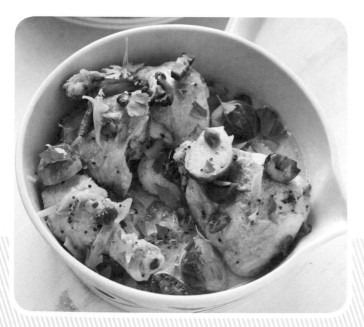

BRUSSELS SPROUTS & LEMON PASTA

SERVES 2

pat of butter
½ tablespoon olive oil
1 small onion, finely diced
3 sprigs of rosemary,
roughly chopped
6 ounces brussels sprouts,
finely shredded
½ cup heavy cream
zest and juice of 1 lemon
7 ounces dried pasta
salt and pepper, to taste
shredded Parmesan, to serve

METHOD

1   Melt the butter and oil in a large skillet. Add the onion and rosemary, season with salt and pepper. Soften over medium–low heat, stirring occasionally, until golden brown.

2   Increase the heat and tip in the sprouts along with 2 tablespoons of water. Cover and cook for 4 minutes, or until the sprouts are tender.

3   Remove the lid, stir in the cream and the lemon zest and juice. Season with salt and pepper.

4   Meanwhile bring a large saucepan of lightly salted water to a boil. Add the pasta, bring back to a boil, and cook according to the package directions, until tender but still firm to the bite. Drain and add to the pan with the sprouts and cream.

5   Toss everything together and divide between warmed bowls. Serve topped with generous handful of shredded Parmesan.

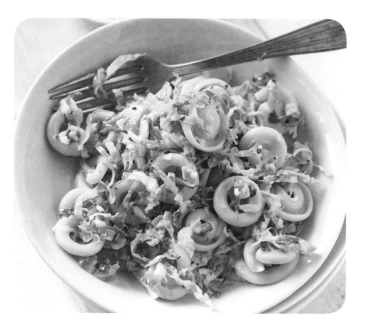

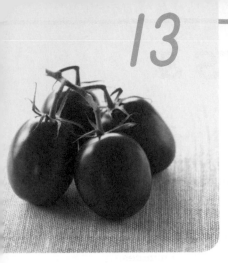

13

TOMATOES

The tomato is one of the healthiest foods because it contains lycopene, which offers protection from prostate cancer, and compounds to help prevent blood clots.

Tomatoes are our major source of dietary lycopene, a carotene antioxidant, that fights heart disease and may help to prevent prostate cancer. Tomatoes also have an anticoagulant effect because of the salicylates contained in them, and they contain several other antioxidants including vitamin C, quercetin, and lutein. Tomatoes are low in calories but high in potassium, and contain useful amounts of fiber.

- Rich source of lycopene, which helps prevent prostate cancer.
- One medium tomato contains nearly one-quarter of the day's recommended intake of vitamin C for an adult.
- Rich in potassium to help regulate body fluids.
- Quercetin and lutein content helps prevent cataracts and keep the heart and eyes healthy.
- Contain salicylates, which have an anticoagulant effect.

Practical tips:
The more red and ripe the tomato, the higher the levels of lycopene contained within it. Vine-ripened tomatoes also contain more lycopene than those ripened after picking. The tomato peel is richer in nutrients than the flesh and the seed part in the center is high in salicylates, so for maximum nutritional benefits, avoid peeling and don't seed unless necessary. The lycopene in raw or cooked tomatoes is better absorbed in your body if it is eaten with some oil, so raw tomatoes are ideally accompanied by a vinaigrette or olive-base dressing.

MAJOR NUTRIENTS PER MEDIUM TOMATO

Calories	18
Total fat	0.2g
Protein	0.9g
Carbohydrate	3.9g
Fiber	1.2g
Vitamin C	12.7mg
Potassium	237mg
Lycopene	2,573mcg
Lutein/Zeaxanthin	123mcg

DID YOU KNOW?

Lycopene is actually more active in processed tomato products, such as ketchup, tomato paste, and tomato juice, than it is in the raw tomato.

TOMATO SAUCE

MAKES 2½ CUPS

1 tablespoon olive oil

1 small onion, chopped

2–3 garlic cloves, crushed

1 small celery stalk,
finely chopped

1 bay leaf

4 ripe tomatoes,
peeled and chopped

1 tablespoon tomato paste,
blended with ½ cup water

few fresh oregano sprigs

pepper, to taste

METHOD

1   Heat the oil in a heavy saucepan over medium heat. Add the onion, garlic, celery, and bay leaf, and cook, stirring frequently, for 5 minutes.

2   Stir in the tomatoes and the tomato paste. Season with pepper and add the oregano. Bring to a boil, then reduce the heat, cover, and simmer, stirring occasionally, for 20–25 minutes, until the tomatoes have completely collapsed. Simmer for an additional 20 minutes to make a thicker sauce, if preferred.

3   Discard the bay leaf and oregano. Transfer to a blender or food processor and process until a chunky puree forms. If a smooth sauce is preferred, pass through a fine nonmetallic strainer. Season with pepper, reheat, and use as required.

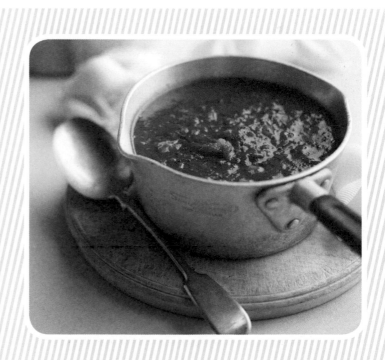

UPSIDE-DOWN TOMATO TART

SERVES 4

2 tablespoons salted butter
1 tablespoon sugar
9 small tomatoes, halved
1 garlic clove, crushed
2 teaspoons white
wine vinegar
salt and pepper, to taste

PIE DOUGH

2 cups all-purpose flour
pinch of salt
1¼ sticks salted butter
1 tablespoon chopped
oregano, plus extra
to garnish
about ⅓ cup cold water

METHOD

1 Preheat the oven to 400°F. To make the filling, melt the butter in a heavy saucepan Add the sugar and stir over high heat until just turning golden brown. Remove from the heat and quickly add the tomatoes, garlic, and white wine vinegar, stirring to coat evenly. Season with salt and pepper.

2 Transfer the tomatoes, cut-side down, to a 9-inch cake pan, spreading them evenly.

3 To make the dough, place the flour, salt, butter, and oregano in a food processor and process until the mixture resembles fine bread crumbs. Add just enough water to bind to a soft, but not sticky, dough. Roll out the dough to a 10-inch circle and put it over the tomatoes, tucking in the edges. Pierce with a fork to let out steam.

4 Bake in the preheated oven for 25–30 minutes, or until firm and golden. Rest for 2–3 minutes, then run a knife around the edge and invert onto a warm serving plate.

5 Sprinkle the tart with chopped oregano, and serve immediately.

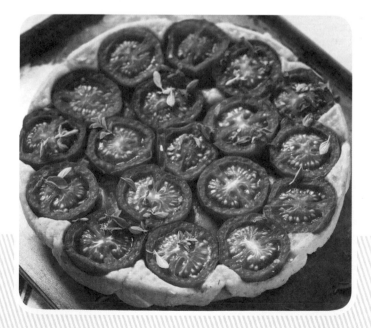

EGGS BAKED IN BEEFSTEAK TOMATOES

MAKES 4

4 large beefsteak tomatoes

4 eggs

2 tablespoons chopped fresh oregano

¼ cup freshly grated Parmesan cheese

1 garlic clove, halved

4 slices sourdough bread or white bread

2 tablespoons olive oil

salt and pepper, to taste

METHOD

1 Preheat the oven to 425°F. Cut a slice from the top of each tomato and scoop out the seeds and pulp. Place the tomatoes in a baking dish or pan.

2 Break an egg into each tomato, then sprinkle with oregano and salt and pepper. Sprinkle with the cheese and bake in the preheated oven for about 20 minutes, or until the eggs are just set, with runny yolks.

3 Meanwhile, rub the garlic over the bread, place on a baking sheet, and drizzle with oil. Bake in the oven for 5–6 minutes, or until golden.

4 Put each egg-filled tomato on a slice of toast and serve immediately.

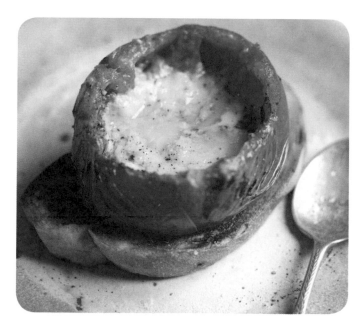

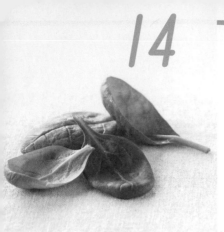

14

SPINACH

Contrary to popular belief, spinach doesn't contain noteworthy levels of iron; nevertheless, it does have many excellent nutritional properties.

Researchers have found that many flavonoid compounds in spinach act as antioxidants and fight against stomach, skin, breast, prostate, and other cancers. Spinach is also extremely high in carotenes, which protect eyesight. It is particularly rich in vitamin K, which helps to boost bone strength and may help prevent osteoporosis. In addition to this, spinach contains peptides, which are aspects of protein that have been shown to lower blood pressure, and its relatively high vitamin E content may help protect the brain from age-related cognitive decline.

• Contains alpha-lipoic acid and glutathione to help retain healthy brain function.
• Source of folate, needed for cell growth, energy, and renewal.
• Contains good levels of essential amino acids, crucial for bone and muscle repair.
• Iron content helps distribute oxygen around the body, which, in turn, is necessary for cell replenishment.

Practical tips:
Avoid buying spinach with any yellowing leaves; in fact, the darker the leaves, the higher the levels of nutrients contained within. The carotenes in spinach are better absorbed when the leaves are cooked compared with when eaten raw, and also if eaten with a little oil. Steaming or stir-frying retains the most antioxidants. To cook, simply wash the leaves and cook in only the water still clinging to the leaves, stirring if necessary.

MAJOR NUTRIENTS PER 3½ CUPS/3½ OUNCES SPINACH

Calories	23
Total fat	0.4g
Protein	2.2g
Carbohydrate	3.6g
Fiber	2.2g
Vitamin C	28mg
Vitamin A	9,377 IU
Beta-carotene	5,626mcg
Vitamin E	2.03mg
Vitamin K	483mg
Folate	194mg
Calcium	99mg
Magnesium	79mg
Iron	2.071mg

DID YOU KNOW?

Spinach contains the chemical tyramine, which increases the release of stimulating brain chemicals. If you don't sleep well, avoid this food close to bedtime.

RED CURRY WITH SPINACH

SERVES 4

2 tablespoons peanut oil or vegetable oil

2 onions, thinly sliced

1 bunch of asparagus spears

1¾ cups reduced-fat coconut milk

2 tablespoons red curry paste

3 fresh kaffir lime leaves

8 cups (about 8 ounces) baby spinach leaves

2 heads bok choy, chopped

1 small head napa cabbage, shredded

handful of fresh cilantro, chopped

cooked rice, to serve

METHOD

1   Heat a wok or skillet over medium–high heat. Add the oil and heat for 30 seconds. Add the onions and asparagus spears and stir-fry for 1–2 minutes.

2   Add the coconut milk, curry paste, and lime leaves and bring gently to a boil. Add the spinach, bok choy, and cabbage and cook for 2–3 minutes, until wilted. Stir in the cilantro and serve with rice.

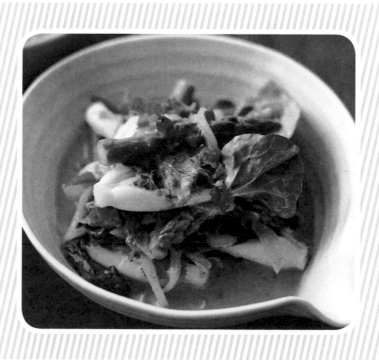

SPINACH & FETA POCKETS

MAKES 6

2 tablespoons olive oil,
plus extra for greasing

1 bunch scallions, chopped

1 pound spinach leaves,
coarsely chopped,
thawed if frozen

1 egg, beaten

1 cup crumbled feta cheese

½ teaspoon freshly
grated nutmeg

6 sheets phyllo pastry

4 tablespoons butter, melted

1 tablespoon sesame seeds

salt and pepper, to taste

METHOD

1 Preheat the oven to 400°F. Grease a baking sheet with oil.

2 Heat the oil in a wok or large skillet, add the scallions, and sauté for 1–2 minutes. Add the spinach and stir until the leaves are wilted. Cook, stirring occasionally, for 2–3 minutes. Drain off any free liquid and let cool slightly.

3 Stir the egg, cheese, and nutmeg into the spinach and season well with salt and pepper.

4 Brush three sheets of pastry with butter. Place another three sheets on top and brush with butter. Cut each sheet down the middle to make six long strips in total. Place a spoonful of the spinach filling on the end of each strip.

5 Lift one corner of pastry over the filling to the opposite side, then turn over the opposite way to enclose. Continue to fold over down the strip to make a triangular pocket, finishing with the seam underneath.

6 Place the pockets on the baking sheet, brush with butter, and sprinkle with the sesame seeds. Bake in the preheated oven for 12–15 minutes, or until golden brown and crisp. Serve.

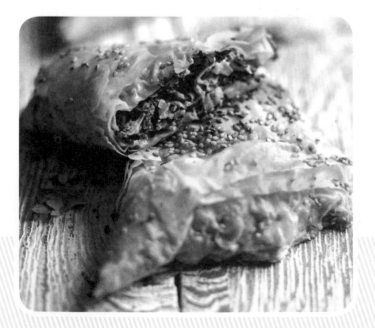

SPINACH & HAM PASTA

SERVES 4

8 ounces dried penne pasta
2 tablespoons olive oil
1 onion, thinly sliced
1 dried red chile, chopped
2 plum tomatoes, diced
8 ounces cooked ham, sliced into strips
1 (8-ounce) package baby spinach leaves
salt and pepper

METHOD

1   Bring a large, heavy saucepan of lightly salted water to a boil. Add the penne, bring back to a boil, and cook according to the package directions, until just tender but still firm to the bite. Drain.

2   Meanwhile, heat the oil in a large skillet over medium heat, add the onion and sauté, stirring, for 2–3 minutes, until soft.

3   Add the chile and tomatoes and cook, stirring, for 2 minutes, then add the ham and cook, stirring, for 2–3 minutes, until heated through.

4   Add the spinach and stir until the leaves are just wilted, then stir in the pasta. Season with salt and pepper and serve.

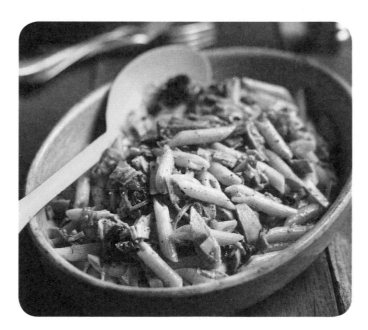

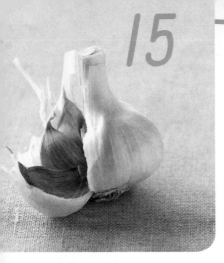

15

GARLIC

Valued as a health protector for thousands of years, garlic bulbs are a useful antibiotic and are also believed to reduce the risk of both heart disease and cancer.

Although often used in only small quantities, garlic can still have a positive effect on health. It contains powerful sulfur compounds, which cause garlic's characteristic strong odor but are also the main source of its health benefits. Research has found that regularly eating garlic could help minimize the risk of heart disease and many types of cancer. It is a powerful antibiotic and inhibits fungal infections, such as athlete's foot. It also appears to minimize stomach ulcers. Eaten in reasonable quantity, garlic is a good source of vitamin C, selenium, potassium, and calcium.

- May prevent formation of blood clots and arterial plaque and as a result prevent heart disease.
- Regular garlic consumption can reduce the risk of colon, stomach, and prostate cancers.
- Naturally antibiotic, antiviral, and antifungal.
- Could help to prevent stomach ulcers.

Practical tips:
Choose large, firm, undamaged garlic bulbs and store in a container with air holes in a dark, cool, dry place. Skin the garlic by lightly crushing the clove with the flat side of a knife and only lightly cook—long cooking destroys its beneficial compounds. Crush or chop garlic and let stand for a few minutes prior to cooking. Eating parsley after a garlic meal may reduce any mouth odor.

MAJOR NUTRIENTS PER 2 GARLIC CLOVES

Calories	9
Total fat	Trace
Protein	0.4g
Carbohydrate	2g
Fiber	Trace
Vitamin C	2mg
Potassium	24mg
Calcium	11mg
Selenium	11mg

DID YOU KNOW?

Cooking meat at high temperatures can have a carcinogenic effect, but when garlic is used with the meat, it reduces the production of the cancer-promoting chemicals.

GARLIC MUSHROOMS

SERVES 4

2 garlic bulbs

2 tablespoons olive oil

12 ounces cremini
mushrooms, halved if large

1 tablespoon chopped
fresh parsley

8 scallions, cut into
1-inch lengths

salt and pepper

METHOD

1   Preheat the oven to 350°F. Separate the garlic bulbs into cloves
    and lightly crush them. Place in an ovenproof dish. Drizzle
    2 teaspoons of the oil over the garlic cloves, season generously
    with salt and pepper, and roast in the preheated oven for
    30 minutes.

2   Remove the garlic from the oven and drizzle with 1 teaspoon
    of the remaining oil. Return to the oven and roast for an
    additional 45 minutes. Remove from the oven and let cool,
    then peel the cloves.

3   Heat a skillet over medium heat. Add the oil from the roasting
    dish, the remaining oil, and the mushrooms to the skillet and
    cook, stirring frequently, for 4 minutes.

4   Add the garlic cloves, parsley, and scallions and cook, stirring
    frequently, for 5 minutes. Season with salt and pepper and
    serve immediately.

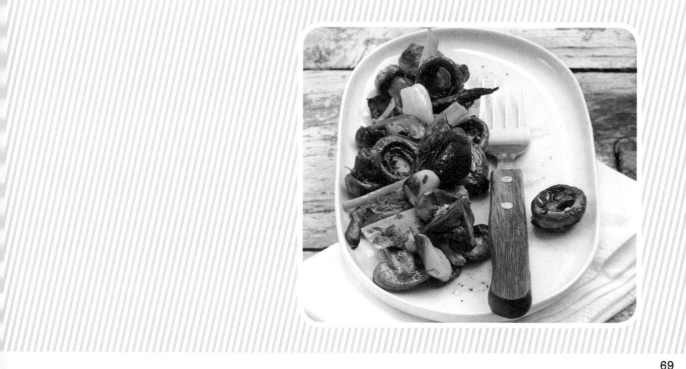

TURKEY STEAK WITH GARLIC & BUTTER BEANS

SERVES 4

1 tablespoon all-purpose flour

1 teaspoon dried thyme

4 turkey cutlets

2 tablespoons olive oil

1 red onion, thinly sliced

4 garlic cloves, crushed

1 cup drained, rinsed canned lima beans

1 (14½ -ounce) can diced tomatoes

salt and pepper, to taste

METHOD

1   Put the flour and thyme into a shallow bowl, season with salt and pepper, and mix. Add the turkey cutlets and turn in the mixture until lightly coated.

2   Heat the oil in a skillet, add the turkey cutlets, and sauté over high heat, turning once, for 2–3 minutes, until golden.

3   Add the onion and garlic and cook for an additional minute, then stir in the beans and tomatoes.

4   Bring to a boil, then reduce the heat, cover the skillet, and simmer gently, stirring occasionally, for 10–15 minutes, until the turkey is tender and no longer pink when cut into with a knife. Season with salt and pepper and serve.

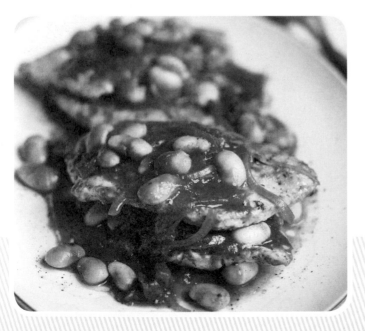

ROASTED GARLIC, SQUASH & THYME SOUP

SERVES 6

¼ cup olive oil, plus extra
for drizzling

2 garlic bulbs

1 butternut squash, peeled,
seeded and cut into
large chunks

2 tablespoons fresh thyme
leaves, plus extra sprigs
to garnish

2 tablespoons butter

1 onion, chopped

1 tablespoon all-purpose flour

5 cups chicken stock

½ cup crème fraîche or
sour cream, to serve

salt and pepper, to taste

METHOD

1   Preheat the oven to 375°F. Pour ½ tablespoon of the oil over
each garlic bulb and season with salt and pepper, then wrap in
aluminum foil and put in a large roasting pan. Toss the squash
in the remaining oil, season with salt and pepper, and sprinkle
with half the thyme leaves. Put in the roasting pan and cook in
the preheated oven for 1 hour.

2   Melt the butter in a large saucepan. Add the onion and cook over
medium heat for 5 minutes, until soft. Stir in the flour and cook,
stirring, for 2 minutes. Add the stock, a few spoonfuls at a time.

3   Add the roasted squash to the saucepan and simmer for
10 minutes.

4   Open the garlic packages and let cool. When cool enough
to handle, squeeze out the garlic pulp from each clove and add
to the soup.

5   Stir in the remaining thyme leaves, then transfer to a food
processor or blender, in batches if necessary, and process
until smooth. Return the soup to the rinsed-out pan and reheat
gently; do not boil. Serve with crème fraîche, garnished with
thyme sprigs.

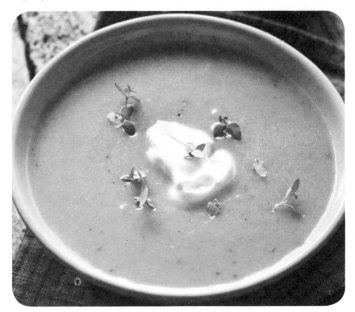

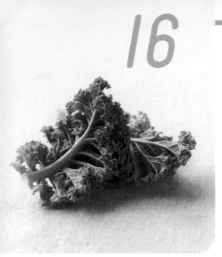

16

KALE

A very nutritious member of the brassica (cabbage) family, kale has the highest levels of antioxidants of all vegetables and is a good source of vitamin C.

Kale is one of the most nutritious members of the brassica family. It is the vegetable with the highest antioxidant capacity, and also contains more calcium and iron than any other vegetable. A single portion contains twice the recommended daily amount of vitamin C, which helps the vegetable's high iron content to be absorbed by the body when ingested. One 1½-cup (3½-ounce) portion also has about one-fifth of the daily calcium requirement for an adult. Kale is rich in selenium, which helps fight cancer, and it contains magnesium and vitamin E for a healthy heart. There are over 45 different flavonoids in kale that combine antioxidant and anti-inflammatory benefits.

- Rich in flavonoids and antioxidants to fight cancers.
- Contains indoles, which can help lower bad cholesterol and prevent cancer.
- Calcium-rich for healthy bones.
- Extremely rich in carotenes to protect eyes.

Practical tips:
Always wash kale before use because the curly leaves may contain grit or soil. Don't discard the outer, deep green leaves—these contain high amounts of beneficial carotenes and indoles. Treat kale as you would cabbage—it is good steamed or stir-fried. It has a strong taste that goes well with bacon, eggs, and cheese. Kale, like spinach, shrinks a lot during cooking, so make sure you add plenty to the pan.

MAJOR NUTRIENTS PER 1½ CUPS /3½ OUNCES CHOPPED KALE

Calories	50
Total fat	0.7g
Protein	3.3g
Carbohydrate	10g
Fiber	2g
Vitamin C	120mg
Folate	29mcg
Vitamin E	1.7mg
Potassium	447mg
Magnesium	34mg
Calcium	135mg
Iron	1.7mg
Selenium	0.9mcg
Beta-carotene	9,226mcg
Lutein/Zeaxanthin	39,550mcg

DID YOU KNOW?

Kale contains naturally occurring substances that can interfere with the functioning of the thyroid glands —people with thyroid problems may not want to eat kale.

RIBOLLITA

SERVES 4

3 tablespoons olive oil
2 red onions, chopped
3 carrots, sliced
3 celery sticks, chopped
3 garlic cloves, chopped
1 tablespoon chopped thyme
1 (14 ounce) can cannellini beans, drained and rinsed
1 (14 ounce) can chopped tomatoes
2 cups vegetable stock
2 tablespoons chopped fresh parsley
1 pound Tuscan kale, trimmed and sliced
1 small day-old ciabatta loaf, torn into small pieces
salt and pepper, to taste

METHOD

1 Heat the oil in a large saucepan and cook the onions, carrots, and celery for 10–15 minutes, stirring frequently. Add the garlic, thyme, and salt and pepper. Continue to cook for a further 1–2 minutes, until the vegetables are golden.

2 Add the cannellini beans to the pan and pour in the tomatoes. Add enough of the stock to cover the vegetables. Bring to the boil and simmer for 20 minutes. Add the parsley and kale and cook for a further 5 minutes. Stir in the bread and add more stock, if needed. The consistency should be thick.

3 Taste and adjust the seasoning, if needed. Ladle into warmed serving bowls and serve hot.

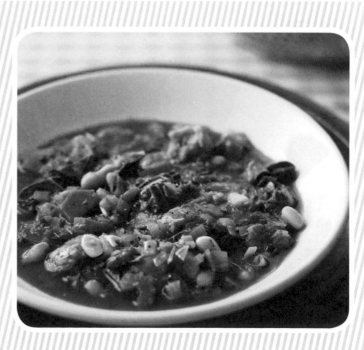

KALE & ARTICHOKE GNOCCHI

SERVES 4

3 cups shredded kale
2 tablespoons olive oil
1 onion, chopped
1 (14-ounce) can artichoke hearts, drained and quartered
2 garlic cloves, chopped
1 teaspoon crushed red pepper flakes
juice of ½ lemon
2 tablespoons pine nuts
salt, to taste

GNOCCHI

6 oven-baked potatoes (about 1½ pounds)
2 cups all-purpose flour, plus extra for dusting
2 tablespoons olive oil

METHOD

1 To make the gnocchi, peel the baked potatoes and mash the flesh until smooth.

2 Turn out the mashed potatoes onto a floured board and knead, working in the flour and oil, for 5 minutes. Divide the mixture into four and roll each into a long sausage shape. Use a knife to cut into pieces about ¾-inch long.

3 Bring a large saucepan of salted water to a boil. Add the kale, return to a boil, and cook for 6–8 minutes. Drain and firmly press out any excess water.

4 Heat the oil in a skillet over high heat. Add the onion and sauté for 3 minutes, then stir in the artichokes, garlic, and red pepper flakes. Cook for 2–3 minutes, then stir in the kale, lemon juice, and pine nuts. Set aside.

5 Bring a large saucepan of salted water to a boil. Add a small batch of the gnocchi, return to a boil, and cook for 2–3 minutes, or until they float on the surface of the water. Cook the remaining batches of the remaining gnocchi in the same way then mix with the kale mixture and serve immediately.

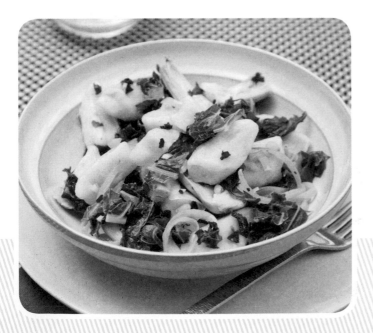

ONE-POT CHICKEN, KALE & CHICKPEA STEW

SERVES 4

1½ tablespoons olive oil

8 chicken thighs

1 large red onion, finely chopped

2 garlic cloves, finely chopped

1 teaspoon red pepper flakes

1 tablespoon tomato paste

1 cup dry white wine

1 cup chicken stock

4 sprigs of thyme

1 (14 ounce) can chopped tomatoes

1 (14 ounce) can chickpeas, drained and rinsed

2¾ ounces kale, shredded

small handful of parsley, leaves chopped

salt and pepper, to taste

METHOD

1 Heat 1 tablespoon of the oil over medium-high heat in a large skillet. Season the chicken generously, add to the pan and brown all over. Remove to a plate.

2 Add the rest of the oil and the onion to the pan, soften for 5 minutes, then add the garlic and red pepper flakes and cook for a couple of minutes more. Stir through the tomato paste, then pour in the wine and stock and bring to a boil.

3 Return the chicken, along with the thyme sprigs, to the pan. Cover and simmer for 10 minutes. Uncover, stir in the tomatoes, and bubble gently for 20 minutes, turning the chicken occasionally.

4 Add the chickpeas and kale, re-cover and cook for 6 minutes or until the chicken is cooked through and the kale is tender. Serve sprinkled with chopped parsley.

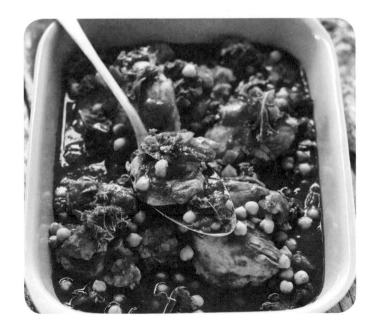

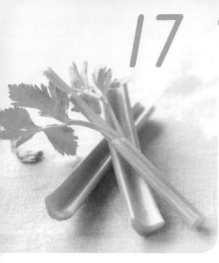

17

CELERY

Typically seen as a dieting snack, celery is high in potassium and calcium, helps reduce fluid retention, and helps prevent high blood pressure.

MAJOR NUTRIENTS PER 2½ STALKS/3½ OUNCES CELERY

Calories	16
Total fat	0.17g
Protein	0.69g
Carbohydrate	2.97g
Fiber	1.6g
Vitamin C	3.1mg
Vitamin B3	0.32mg
Vitamin B5	0.25mg
Folate	36mg
Calcium	40mg
Magnesium	11mg
Potassium	260mg

Celery has long been regarded as an ideal food for dieters because of its high water content and resulting low calorie content. In fact, celery is a useful and healthy vegetable for many other reasons—it is also a good source of potassium and is surprisingly high in calcium, which is vital for healthy bones, healthy blood-pressure levels, and nerve function. The darker-green stalks and the leaves of celery contain higher levels of vitamins and minerals than the paler leaves, so don't discard them. Celery also contains the compounds polyacetylenes and phthalides, which may protect us from inflammation and high blood pressure.

• Low in calories and fat and high in fiber.
• Good source of potassium.
• Calcium content protects bones and may help regulate blood pressure.
• May offer protection from inflammation.

Practical tips:
Choose celery heads with leaves that look bright-green and fresh. Store in a plastic bag or in plastic wrap to prevent the stalks from turning limp. Celery is ideal for adding flavor and bulk to soups and stews and the stalks can be braised in vegetable stock for an excellent accompaniment to fish, poultry, or game. The leaves can be added to salads and stir-fries or used as a garnish.

CELERY & APPLE REVITALIZER

SERVES 2

3 celery stalks, chopped

1 Red Delicious or other crisp apple, peeled, cored, and diced

2½ cups low-fat milk

pinch of sugar (optional)

salt, to taste

METHOD

1 Put the celery, apple, and milk in a blender and process until thoroughly combined.

2 Stir in the sugar, if using, and season with salt. Pour into chilled glasses and serve.

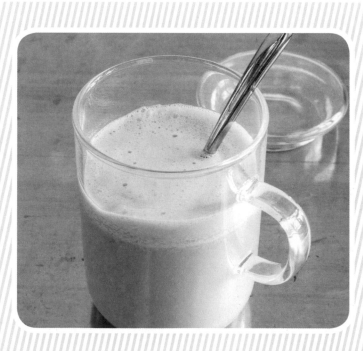

RROT, CELERY & APPLE SOUP

SERVES 4

15 carrots (about 2 pounds), finely diced

1 onion, chopped

3 celery stalks, diced

4 cups vegetable stock

2 Pippin or Gala apples

2 tablespoons tomato paste

1 bay leaf

salt and pepper, to taste

TO GARNISH

1 medium Pippin or Gala apple, thinly sliced

juice of ½ lemon

shredded celery leaves

METHOD

1 Put the carrots, onion, and celery in a large saucepan and add the stock. Bring to a boil, reduce the heat, cover, and simmer for 10 minutes.

2 Meanwhile, peel, core, and dice the apples. Add the diced apple, tomato paste, and bay leaf to the saucepan and bring to a boil over medium heat. Reduce the heat, cover, and simmer for 20 minutes. Remove and discard the bay leaf.

3 Meanwhile, to make the garnish, put the apple slices in a small saucepan and pour the lemon juice over the slices. Heat the apple slices gently and simmer for 1–2 minutes, or until the apple is tender. Drain the apple slices and reserve until required.

4 Transfer the carrot-and-apple mixture to a food processor or blender, in batches if necessary, and process until smooth. Return the soup to the rinsed-out saucepan, reheat gently, and season with salt and pepper. Ladle the soup into warm bowls, top with the reserved apple slices and shredded celery leaves, and serve immediately.

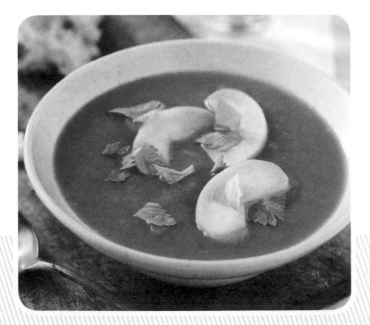

MARINATED BEEF WITH CELERY

SERVES 4

1 pound 2 ounces beef tenderloin, cut into thin strips

1 cup vegetable oil

3 celery stalks, cut into long 1-inch-thick strips

1 red bell pepper, cut into thin strips

1 red chile, seeded and finely sliced

lime wedges, to garnish

cooked rice and Thai fish sauce, to serve

MARINADE

1 teaspoon salt

2 tablespoons Thai fish sauce

METHOD

1 To make the marinade, mix the salt and fish sauce in a large bowl.

2 Add the beef and toss to coat. Cover with plastic wrap and put in the refrigerator for 1 hour to marinate.

3 Heat a wok over medium heat, then add the oil and heat to 350–375°F, or until a cube of bread browns in 30 seconds. Add the beef and deep-fry for 2–3 minutes, or until crispy. Remove the wok from the heat and, using a slotted spoon, lift out the meat and drain it on paper towels. Discard all but 2 tablespoons of the oil.

4 Reheat the reserved oil in the wok, add the celery, bell pepper, and chile, and stir-fry for 1 minute. Add the beef and cook, until hot.

5 Garnish with lime wedges and serve immediately with rice and fish sauce.

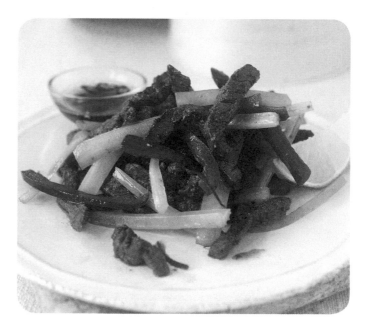

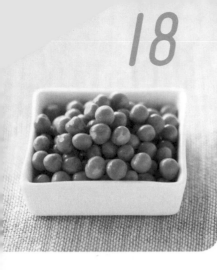

18

PEAS

Whether freshly picked or bought frozen, peas are packed with vitamin C, are a rich source of fiber, and also contain lutein, which is important for healthy eyes.

MAJOR NUTRIENTS PER ⅔ CUP/3½ OUNCES SHELLED PEAS

Calories	81
Total fat	0.4g
Protein	5.4g
Carbohydrate	14.5g
Fiber	5.1g
Vitamin C	40mg
Vitamin E	Trace
Folate	65mcg
Potassium	244mg
Lutein/Zeaxanthin	2,477mcg

Peas are rich in a wide range of useful vitamins and minerals. They are particularly high in antioxidants, such as vitamin C, folate, and vitamin B3, and their very high lutein and zeaxanthin content means that they help protect the eyes from macular degeneration. The B vitamins they contain may help protect the bones from osteoporosis, and they may help to decrease the risk of strokes by keeping levels of the amino acid homocysteine low in the blood. Peas are also an important source of protein for those on restricted diets, such as vegetarians. In addition, their high fiber content partly comprises pectin, a jellylike substance that helps to lower bad blood cholesterol and may also help prevent heart and arterial disease.

• Contain several heart-friendly nutrients and chemicals.
• Rich in carotenes to protect eyes and reduce risk of cancers.
• High in total and soluble fiber, which could lower cholesterol.
• Very rich in vitamin C.

Practical tips:
When buying peas in the pod, choose those that aren't packed in too tightly. Older peas become almost square, lose their flavor, and become mealy because the sugars have been converted to starches. Young pods can be eaten with the peas inside and young peas can be eaten raw. To cook, steam lightly or boil in minimal water, because the vitamin C content diminishes in water.

DID YOU KNOW?

Frozen peas can often contain more vitamin C and other nutrients than fresh peas in their pods, which may be several days old.

CHILLED PEA SOUP

SERVES 4

2 cups vegetable stock
or water
3 cups frozen peas
3 scallions, coarsely chopped
1¼ cups plain yogurt
salt and pepper, to taste

TO GARNISH

2 tablespoons chopped
fresh mint
grated lemon rind
olive oil

METHOD

1   Bring the stock to a boil in a large saucepan over medium heat. Reduce the heat, add the peas and scallions, and simmer for 5 minutes.

2   Let cool slightly, then blend until smooth using a handheld immersion blender or a food processor. Pour into a large bowl, season with salt and pepper, and stir in the yogurt. Cover the bowl with plastic wrap and chill in the refrigerator for several hours, or until well chilled.

3   To serve, remove from the refrigerator, mix well, and ladle into soup bowls. Garnish with the chopped mint, grated lemon rind, and a drizzle of olive oil.

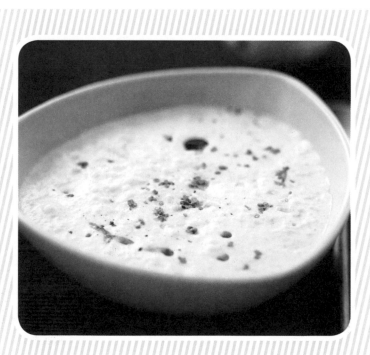

PEAS WITH LETTUCE

SERVES 4–6

2 tablespoons salted butter, plus an extra pat

1 teaspoon sunflower oil

1 ounce unsmoked bacon, chopped

1 shallot, finely chopped

2 cups shelled peas

1¼ cups vegetable stock or water

1 Boston lettuce or butter lettuce, cored and shredded

2 tablespoons chopped fresh chervil

salt and pepper

METHOD

1   Melt the butter with the oil in a large saucepan over medium heat. Add the bacon and stir for 3 minutes. Add the shallot and continue sautéing for another 3 minutes.

2   Add the peas and stock and season with salt and pepper (but remember that the bacon will be salty). Cover the pan and bring to a boil over high heat, then uncover, reduce the heat slightly, and simmer for 5 minutes.

3   Add the lettuce and continue to simmer, uncovered, until the peas are tender and the liquid has evaporated. Stir in the pat of butter, then taste and adjust the seasoning with salt and pepper, if necessary. Stir in the chervil and serve immediately.

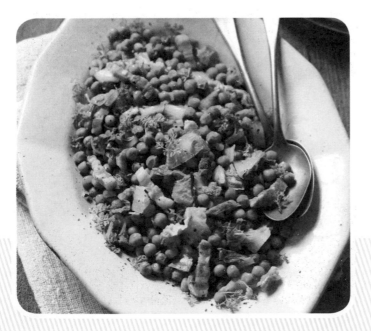

PEA & MINT RISOTTO

SERVES 4

2 tablespoons olive oil
3 tablespoons butter
1 onion, finely chopped
1 garlic clove, crushed
2 cups risotto rice
⅔ cup dry white wine
6½ cups boiling chicken stock
or vegetable stock
3 cups fresh or frozen peas
2 tablespoons chopped
fresh mint
salt and pepper

METHOD

1 Heat the oil with 1 tablespoon of the butter in a large, heavy saucepan. Add the onion and sauté gently over medium heat, stirring, for 4–5 minutes, until soft but not brown.

2 Add the garlic and rice and cook, stirring, for 1–2 minutes. Stir in the wine, bring to a boil, and cook, stirring, for about 1 minute.

3 Gradually add the stock, stirring until each addition is absorbed before adding the next. Stir in the peas and half the mint with the final addition of stock.

4 Continue stirring until most of the liquid has been absorbed and the rice is almost tender, with a slight firmness in the center. Stir in the remaining butter.

5 Season with salt and pepper, stir in the remaining mint, and serve.

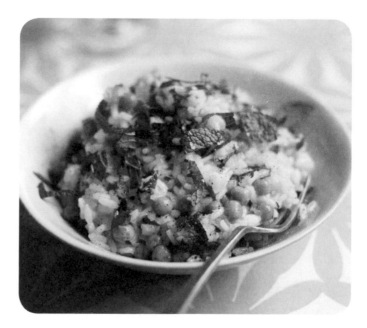

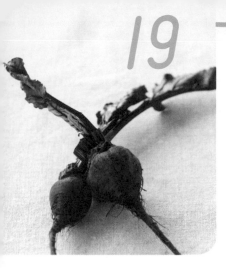

BEETS

These colorful, sweet roots may not be the richest vegetable in nutrients, but they certainly should not be overlooked and are invaluable during the winter season.

MAJOR NUTRIENTS PER 1¼ CUPS/3½ OUNCES BEETS

Calories	36
Total fat	**Trace**
Protein	**1.7g**
Carbohydrate	**7.6g**
Fiber	**1.9g**
Vitamin C	**5mg**
Folate	**150mg**
Potassium	**380mg**
Calcium	**20mg**
Iron	**1.0mg**
Magnesium	**23mg**

Beets come in white and gold varieties as well as the classic purple-red, which is the best source of nutrients. Betaine, which gives them their deep color, is even more potent an antioxidant than polyphenols in its effect on lowering blood pressure. A scientific study also found that the high levels of nitrates in beet juice work like aspirin to prevent blood clots, and help to protect the lining of the blood vessels. Red beets are also rich in anthocyanins, which may help to prevent colon and other cancers.

• Betaine helps lower blood pressure and has anti-inflammatory properties.
• Contain nitrates, which help prevent blood clots.
• Anthocyanins can help prevent cancers.
• A good source of iron, magnesium, and folate.

Practical tips:
Cooked beets will keep in an airtight container in the refrigerator for a few days, or you can puree cooked beets and freeze them. To cook, cut off the leaves so that about 2 inches of stems remain, and keep the root in place. This will prevent the beets from "bleeding" as they cook. Beets can be boiled whole for about 50 minutes or brushed with a little oil and baked in aluminum foil at 400°F for 1 hour. The skins can then be easily rubbed off. Beets can also be used raw, peeled and shredded into salads or salsa, or juiced.

BEET & SPINACH SALAD

SERVES 4

3 tablespoons extra virgin olive oil

juice of 1 orange

1 teaspoon sugar

1 teaspoon fennel seeds

5 cups diced, cooked beets

1 (4-ounce) package fresh baby spinach leaves

salt and pepper, or to taste

METHOD

1 Heat the olive oil in a small, heavy saucepan. Add the orange juice, sugar, and fennel seeds and season with salt and pepper. Stir continuously until the sugar has dissolved.

2 Add the beets to the saucepan and stir gently to coat. Remove from the heat.

3 Arrange the spinach leaves in a large salad bowl. Spoon the warm beets on top and serve immediately.

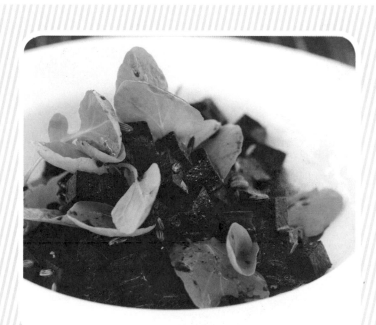

BEET BURGER

MAKES 4

½ cup millet
¾ cup lightly salted water
1 cup grated raw beets
(from 1–2 beets)
½ cup grated carrot
½ cup grated zucchini
½ cup finely chopped walnuts
2 tablespoons cider vinegar
2 tablespoons extra virgin
olive oil, plus extra
for frying
salt and pepper
1 egg
2 tablespoons cornstarch
4 multigrain buns, halved
lettuce leaves

METHOD

1   Rinse and drain the millet, then put it into in a small saucepan
with the salted water. Place over medium heat, bring to a
simmer, cover, and cook over low heat for 20–25 minutes.
Remove from the heat and let stand for 5 minutes, covered.

2   Put the beet, carrot, zucchini, and walnuts into a large bowl. Add
the millet, vinegar, oil, ½ teaspoon of salt, and ¼ teaspoon of
pepper and mix well. Add the egg and cornstarch, mix again,
then chill in the refrigerator for 2 hours.

3   Pack the beet mixture into a ½ cup measure, then shape into a
patty. Repeat to make a total of four patties. Place a griddle or
large skillet over medium heat and coat with oil. Add the patties
and cook for about 5 minutes on each side, turning carefully,
until brown.

4   To serve, place the burgers in the buns, topped with the lettuce.
Serve immediately.

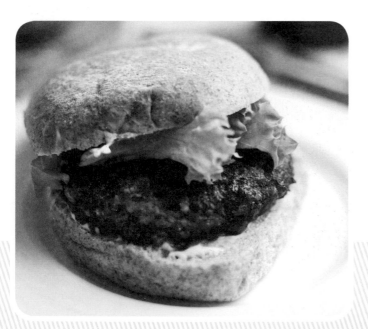

BEET RISOTTO

SERVES 6

6 raw, whole beets, unpeeled
2 tablespoons olive oil
1 onion, finely chopped
1 garlic clove, finely chopped
1⅓ cups risotto rice
3⅓ cups vegetable stock
1 cup dry white wine
salt and pepper, to taste

TOPPING

1 tablespoon caraway seeds
1 cup fresh white
bread crumbs
½ teaspoon granulated sugar
1 tablespoon vegetable oil

METHOD

1 Place the beets in a large saucepan, cover with water, and bring to a boil. Cook for 45 minutes, or until the beets are soft. Drain in a colander and peel the beets under cold running water. Trim away any remaining skin with a knife and set aside.

2 Preheat the oven to 350°F. Heat the oil in a large ovenproof casserole dish over medium heat. Sauté the onion and garlic for 3–4 minutes, or until soft. Stir in the rice, stock, and ⅔ cup of the wine, cover, and transfer to the preheated oven. Cook for 30 minutes, until the rice is tender.

3 To make the topping, crush the caraway seeds and then mix all the topping ingredients together in a small bowl. Transfer to a small skillet and sauté, stirring continuously, over medium heat for 2–3 minutes. Transfer to a plate to cool.

4 Process one-quarter of the beets to a smooth puree in a food processor. Chop the remaining beets finely. Stir the chopped and pureed beets into the risotto along with the remaining wine, and season with salt and pepper. To serve, divide among serving plates and sprinkle with the topping.

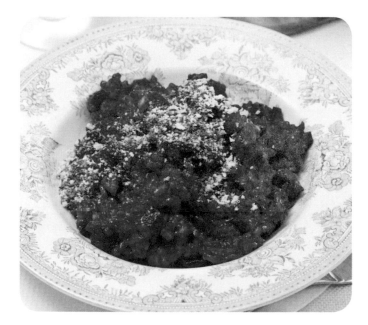

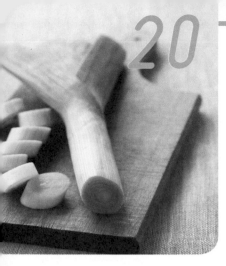

20

LEEKS

Members of the health-giving allium family, along with garlic and onions, leeks contain a combination of nutrients for healthy skin, bones, and heart.

MAJOR NUTRIENTS PER AVERAGE LEEK

Calories	61
Total fat	0.3g
Protein	1.5g
Carbohydrate	2.9g
Fiber	1.8g
Vitamin C	12mg
Vitamin B6	0.23mg
Vitamin K	47mcg
Folate	64mcg
Calcium	59mcg
Magnesium	28mg

Leeks have a distinct, slightly sweet, onion flavor but are milder than most onions. The long, thick stems have a lower white area and dark green tops, which are edible but are usually removed because they can be tough. Leeks have been shown to reduce total bad blood cholesterol while raising good cholesterol, and so can help to prevent heart and arterial disease. Regular consumption is also linked with a reduction in the risk of prostate, ovarian, and colon cancers. It is the allylic sulfides in the plants that appear to confer these cancer-fighting benefits, but they are also rich in vitamin C, fiber, vitamin E, folate, and several important minerals.

- Lower total bad cholesterol levels in the blood and raise good cholesterol.
- Mildly diuretic to help prevent fluid retention.
- High in carotenes, including lutein and zeaxanthin, for eye health.

Practical tips:
Wash leeks thoroughly before using—they may contain soil between the tight leaves. The more of the green section of the leek that you use, the more of the beneficial nutrients you will retain. Instead of boiling, steam, bake, or stir-fry leeks to retain their vitamins. The darker-green parts take a little longer to cook than the white part, so, if chopped, add the green parts to the pan first.

88

LEEK & POTATO SOUP

SERVES 4–6

2 tablespoons butter

1 onion, chopped

3 leeks, sliced

8 ounces Yukon gold potatoes, peeled and cut into ¾-inch cubes

3½ cups vegetable stock

salt and pepper, to taste

½ cup light cream (optional) and 2 tablespoons snipped fresh chives, to garnish

METHOD

1 Melt the butter in a large saucepan over a medium heat, add the vegetables and sauté gently for 2–3 minutes, until soft but not brown. Pour in the stock, bring to a boil, then reduce the heat and simmer, covered, for 15 minutes.

2 Remove from the heat and blend the soup in the saucepan using a hand-held immersion blender if you have one. Otherwise, pour into a blender, blend until smooth and return to the rinsed-out saucepan.

3 Heat the soup, season to taste with salt and pepper and serve in warmed bowls, swirled with the cream, if using, and garnished with chives.

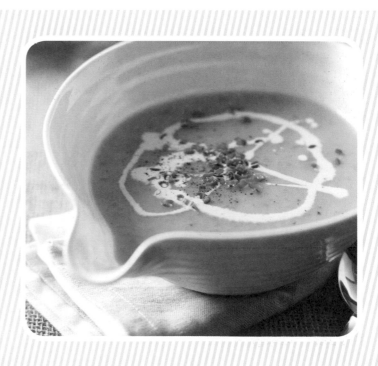

ROASTED LEEKS WITH PARSLEY

SERVES 4

4 large leeks, trimmed and halved lengthwise

3 tablespoons extra virgin olive oil

salt and pepper, to taste

1 tablespoon chopped fresh flat-leaf parsley

METHOD

1 Preheat the oven to 475°F. Pack the leeks in a single layer in a shallow casserole dish.

2 Brush with the olive oil, making sure it goes into the crevices. Season with salt and pepper and sprinkle with the parsley, turning to coat.

3 Roast in the preheated oven for 15–20 minutes, turning once, until the leeks begin to blacken at the edges.
   Serve immediately.

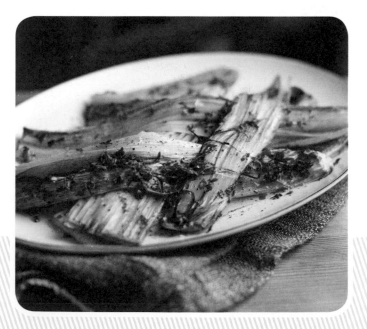

HAM & LEEK CRÊPES

SERVES 2

4 savory crêpes
4 thin slices honey-baked ham
¼ cup shredded Gruyère
cheese

FILLING
2 tablespoons butter
1 tablespoon olive oil
3 leeks, halved, rinsed and
finely shredded
3 shallots, finely chopped
1 teaspoon fresh sage,
finely chopped
2 tablespoons white
wine or water
2 tablespoons heavy cream
salt and pepper, to taste

METHOD

1 To make the filling, heat the butter and oil together in a
saucepan. Add the leeks, shallots, and sage and season with salt
and pepper. Cook, covered, over a low heat for 5 minutes. Add
the wine and cook for 5 minutes more, or until the leeks are
tender. Stir in the cream and remove from the heat.

2 Preheat the oven to 400°F. Lay the crêpes on a work surface and
place a slice of ham on each. Divide the leek mixture among
the crêpes and roll up the crêpes.

3 Transfer to a baking dish and sprinkle the top of each one with
a little grated cheese. Bake in the preheated oven for
15–20 minutes, or until golden and bubbling. Transfer to plates
and serve immediately.

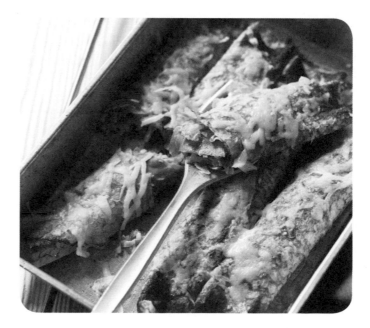

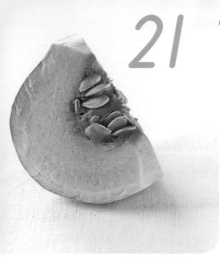

21

PUMPKIN

Pumpkins contain the orange nutrients alpha- and beta-carotene and lutein, powerful anti-aging nutrients that protect your skin against damage from sunlight.

The fat-soluble carotenoids contained in pumpkin are needed to protect fatty areas in the skin, heart, eyes, brain, and liver. As a winter vegetable, pumpkin is well placed to protect the body when it is most needed—we eat more fat in the winter and lay down more fat stores for insulation. The seeds of the pumpkin are incredibly nutrient-rich, while the orange flesh contains malic acid—also found in apples and plums—that is needed by every cell in the body for renewal. In combination with the protective carotenoids, malic acid helps to keep skin firm, bones strong, and vital organs healthy.

- Contains phytosterols, needed for immune function and cholesterol regulation.
- Contains vitamin B2 to activate folate, and vitamin B6 to process fats and proteins from food to repair and rejuvenate body tissues and mucous membranes.

Practical tips:
Like most squash, pumpkin can be boiled, steamed, baked, or roasted, and it can be used to make both sweet desserts and unsweetened dishes. Pumpkin is sometimes oversweetened, which masks its delicate flavor. Try roasting your own pumpkin seeds in the oven for a healthy snack.

MAJOR NUTRIENTS PER 1 CUP/3½ OUNCES PUMPKIN

Calories	13
Total fat	0.1g
Protein	1g
Carbohydrate	6.5g
Fiber	0.5g
Vitamin C	9mg
Vitamin E	1.06mg
Vitamin B2	0.11mg
Vitamin B6	0.06mg
Folate	16mcg
Beta-carotene	3,100mcg
Lutein/Zeaxanthin	1,500mcg
Phytosterols	12mg

DID YOU KNOW?

The name "pumpkin" originally comes from the Greek *peponi*, meaning "large melon." The French called it *pompon*, and the British opted for *pumpion*, before the American name came about.

PUMPKIN RAVIOLI

SERVES 4

store-bought fresh
pasta sheets
semolina flour, for dusting

FILLING
1 tablespoon olive oil
4 cups diced pumpkin
(½-inch pieces)
1 shallot, finely diced
½ cup water, plus extra
for brushing
⅔ cup grated Parmesan
cheese
1 egg
1 tablespoon finely chopped
fresh parsley
salt and pepper, to taste

METHOD

1   To make the filling, heat the olive oil in a saucepan, add the pumpkin and shallot, and sauté for 2–3 minutes, or until the shallot is translucent. Add the water and cook the pumpkin for 15–20 minutes, or until the liquid evaporates. Cool slightly, then mix with the cheese, egg, and parsley. Season with salt and pepper.

2   Dust the counter with semolina flour. Cut the pasta sheet in two. Place small spoonfuls of the pumpkin mixture about 1½ inches apart on one sheet of dough. Brush a little water on the spaces in between. Lay the second sheet of pasta on top and press down around each piece of filling.

3   Use a pastry wheel to cut out squares and press the edges together with a fork. Then bring a large saucepan of lightly salted water to a boil. Add the ravioli, bring back to a boil, and cook over medium heat for 3–4 minutes, or according to the package directions, until tender, but still firm to the bite. Drain the ravioli and serve immediately.

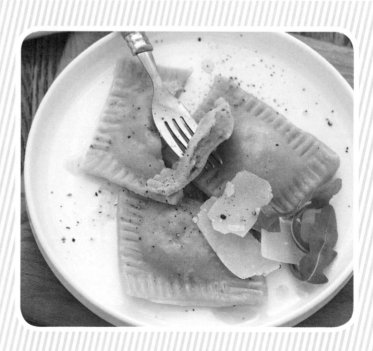

SPICED PUMPKIN TARTLETS

SERVES 4

3 cups diced pumpkin
(½-inch pieces)

1½ teaspoons butter, melted,
plus extra for greasing

1 tablespoon maple syrup

1 piece preserved ginger in
syrup, finely chopped

¼ teaspoon cinnamon

¼ teaspoon allspice

8 sheets phyllo pastry

2 tablespoons canola oil

confectioners' sugar, to serve

METHOD

1   Preheat the oven to 375°F. Lightly grease four 4-inch tart pans.

2   Put the pumpkin on a baking sheet and dot with the butter.
    Roast in the preheated oven for 5 minutes, then stir and return
    to the oven for an additional 20 minutes, or until the pumpkin is
    beginning to brown. Stir in the maple syrup, chopped ginger,
    cinnamon, and allspice, and cook for an additional 5 minutes.
    Let cool.

3   Cut the phyllo pastry into twelve 4-inch squares. Brush four with
    canola oil. Place a second sheet of pastry on top of each, at an
    angle to the first so that the points of the squares do not align—
    creating a star shape. Brush with oil again and finish with the
    remaining pastry sheets to make four stacks, each with three
    layers. Transfer the pastry to the prepared tart pans, press down
    gently, and bake for 8–10 minutes, or until crisp and golden.

4   Fill the pastry shells with the pumpkin mixture. Dust with
    confectioners' sugar and serve immediately.

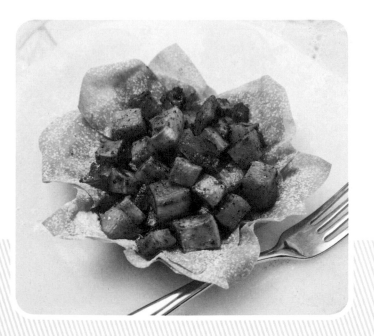

PUMPKIN & SUN-DRIED TOMATO SPAGHETTI

SERVES 4

3 cups diced pumpkin
(½-inch pieces)
2 red onions, cut into wedges
1 tablespoon olive oil
15 sun-dried tomatoes in oil
12 ounces dried spaghetti
salt and pepper, to taste
fresh basil leaves, to garnish

METHOD

1   Preheat the oven to 350°F.
2   Toss the pumpkin and onion together with the olive oil.
    Put in a roasting pan and roast in the preheated oven for 25–30
    minutes, or until tender. Let cool for 5 minutes.
3   Cut the sun-dried tomatoes into small pieces and stir into the
    roasted vegetables. Season with salt and pepper.
4   Bring a large saucepan of salted water to a boil. Add the
    spaghetti, return to a boil, and cook for 8–10 minutes, or until
    tender but still firm to the bite.
5   Drain the spaghetti well and divide among four warm serving
    plates. Top with the vegetables and garnish with fresh basil
    leaves. Serve immediately.

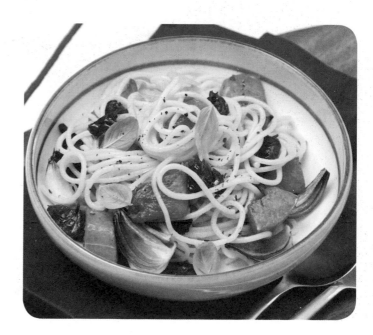

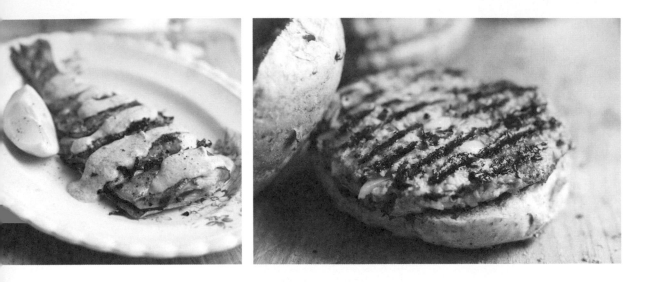

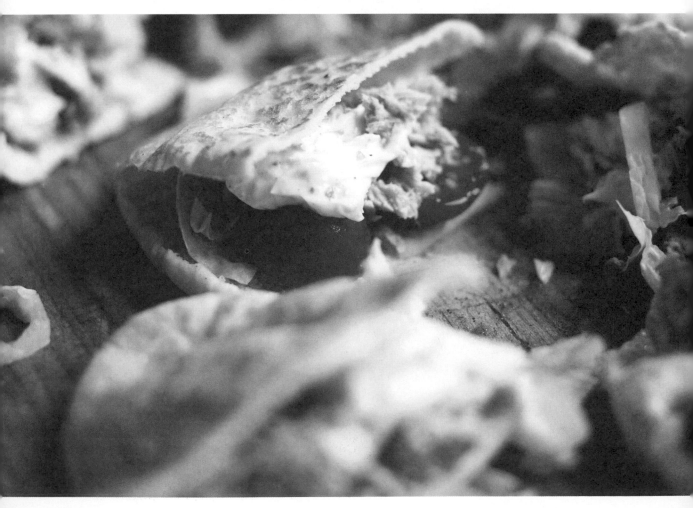

MEAT, POULTRY, FISH & SEAFOOD

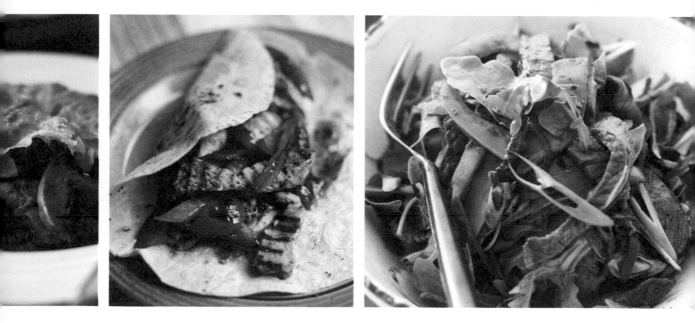

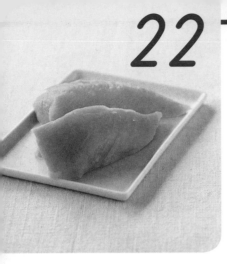

22

TURKEY

A low-fat, high-protein source, turkey is a versatile alternative to chicken—quick and easy to prepare, it's easy to incorporate into the modern diet.

MAJOR NUTRIENTS PER 3½ OUNCES TURKEY, SKIN REMOVED

Calories	111
Total fat	0.65g
Saturated fat	0.21g
Monounsaturated fat	0.11g
Protein	24.6g
Carbohydrate	0mg
Fiber	0mg
Vitamin B3	6.23mg
Vitamin B5	0.72mg
Vitamin B6	0.58mg
Iron	1.17mg
Zinc	1.24mg
Glutamic acid	4.02g

Turkey contains high amounts of tryptophan, a protein constituent that controls both mood and sleep, as well as the neurotransmitter serotonin, which also affects mood and appetite. Turkey's high protein content also helps control appetite by balancing blood-sugar concentration, thus curbing sugar cravings and energy fluctuations. The white meat of turkey is considered healthier than the brown meat due to its lower fat content, but the difference is small. In fact, the brown meat can actually help raise your metabolism more, making you more efficient at burning fuel, more likely to lose weight, and less susceptible to overeating.

- Iron supports energy levels by producing the cells that your body uses for fuel and helping muscles store rejuvenating oxygen.
- Glutamic acid helps balance blood-sugar levels.
- Contains the zinc that is needed to make serotonin, which makes you feel good. It is also vital in the process of repair to the body.

Practical tips:
Turkey can be a lower-fat alternative to chicken, with many similar health benefits. A pasture-raised bird that has had a healthy diet itself and lived more naturally will be leaner, taste better, and lose less water when cooked. Prepare and cook in the same way as you would chicken.

TURKEY SALAD PITA BREAD

SERVES 1

small handful of baby spinach,
rinsed, patted dry,
and shredded

½ red bell pepper, seeded
and thinly sliced

½ carrot, peeled and
grated

¼ cup hummus

⅔ cup thinly sliced, cooked
boneless, skinless turkey

½ tablespoon sunflower
seeds

1 whole-wheat pita bread

salt and pepper, to taste

METHOD

1   Preheat the broiler to medium-high.

2   Put the spinach, red bell pepper, carrot, and hummus into a
large bowl and stir together, so that all the salad ingredients are
coated with the hummus. Stir in the turkey and sunflower seeds
and season with salt and pepper.

3   Put the pita bread under the broiler for about 1 minute on each
side to warm through, but do not brown. Cut it in half to make
two "pockets" of bread.

4   Divide the salad between the bread pockets and serve.

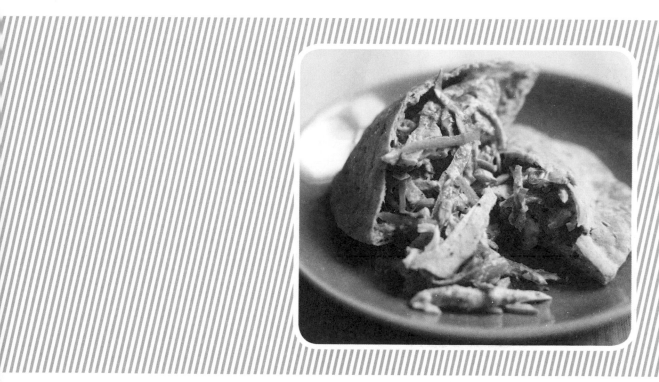

CLASSIC TURKEY BURGER

MAKES 4

12 ounces fresh ground turkey

¼ cup fresh whole-wheat bread crumbs

1 small onion, finely chopped

1 apple, such as McIntosh, peeled, cored, and finely grated

grated rind and juice of 1 small lemon

2 tablespoons finely chopped fresh parsley

sunflower oil, for brushing

salt and pepper, to taste

4 whole-grain sandwich buns or focaccia, halved

METHOD

1   Preheat the broiler to medium-high and line the broiler pan with aluminum foil. Place the turkey, bread crumbs, onion, apple, lemon rind and juice, and parsley into a large bowl. Season with salt and pepper and gently mix to combine. Divide into four equal portions and shape each portion into a patty.

2   Brush the patties with oil and place on the prepared pan. Cook, turning once, for 5 minutes, or until cooked through. To test the burgers, pierce them with the tip of a sharp knife; if the juices run clear, they are ready. If there are any traces of pink, return them to the broiler for 1–2 minutes.

3   Place a burger on each bun bottom, add the bun lids, and serve immediately.

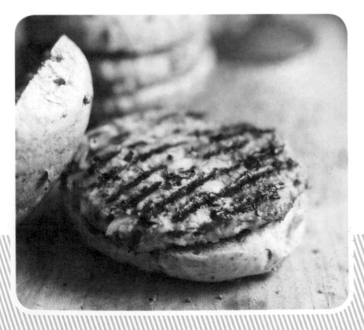

TURKEY CUTLETS WITH TARRAGON SAUCE

SERVES 4

1 tablespoon all-purpose flour

4 turkey cutlets

1 tablespoon olive oil

2 tablespoons butter

2 shallots, finely chopped

⅔ cup dry white wine

thinly pared rind and juice
of ½ lemon

2 tablespoons chopped
fresh tarragon

¼ cup heavy cream

salt and pepper, to taste

METHOD

1 Put the flour into a shallow bowl and season with salt and pepper. Add the turkey cutlets and turn in the flour until lightly coated.

2 Heat the oil with half the butter in a skillet, add the turkey cutlets, and cook over medium heat, turning once, for 8–10 minutes, until golden brown and cooked through. Remove from the skillet and keep warm.

3 Add the remaining butter to the skillet, then add the shallots and sauté, stirring, for 3–4 minutes, until soft. Add the wine, lemon rind and juice, and half the tarragon. Bring to a boil and boil for 2–3 minutes, until reduced by about half.

4 Strain the sauce into a clean saucepan, add the cream and the remaining tarragon, and cook, stirring, until boiling. Adjust the seasoning, then spoon the sauce over the turkey cutlets and serve.

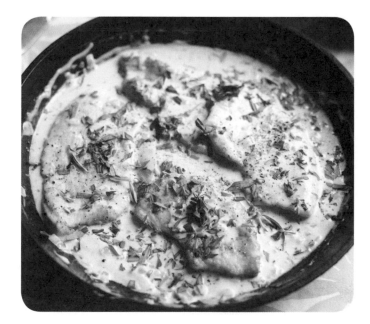

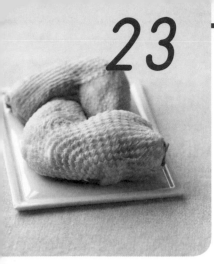

23

CHICKEN

A single serving of protein-rich, pasture-raised chicken provides two-thirds of the nutrients needed by the body to replenish skin, bone, and muscle.

*MAJOR NUTRIENTS
PER 3½ OUNCES CHICKEN,
SKIN REMOVED*

Calories	114
Total fat	2.59g
Saturated fat	0.57g
Monounsaturated fat	0.76g
Protein	21.23g
Carbohydrate	0mg
Fiber	0mg
Vitamin B3	10.43mg
Vitamin B5	1.43mcg
Vitamin B6	0.75mg
Selenium	32mcg
Glutamic acid	3.15g

The human body consists of 22 percent protein, and just under half of this is muscle. Your muscles need continual replenishment, especially after exercise, in order for the body to maintain mobility and posture. Stress uses up protein in the body to make adrenaline, but protein-rich foods such as chicken, in the diet can replace it in a way that the body finds easy to absorb. Chicken that has been reared in a healthy, pasture-raised environment can also provide the B vitamins needed to maintain energy levels and good brain function.

• Protein makes collagen, which is needed on a daily basis to rejuvenate skin, hair, nails, and the internal organs.
• Contains hyaluronic acid, which holds water in collagen in order to keep the body hydrated.
• Contains glutamic acid, the main protein in human muscle, which provides strength and rapid regeneration.
• The antioxidant mineral selenium helps combat toxic metals, such as mercury, lead, and aluminum.

Practical tips:
Choose your chicken wisely—birds raised in confined spaces will not have used their muscles enough to develop as a source of protein and can also be much higher in fat than pasture-raised birds. Although it is a more expensive option, organic chicken is better quality and worth the extra cost.

THAI CHICKEN

SERVES 4

6 garlic cloves,
coarsely chopped

1 teaspoon pepper

8 chicken legs

1 tablespoon Thai fish sauce

¼ cup dark soy sauce

fresh ginger, cut into
matchsticks, to garnish

METHOD

1   Put the garlic in a mortar. Add the pepper, and pound to a paste with a pestle. Using a sharp knife, make three to four diagonal slashes on both sides of each chicken leg. Spread the garlic paste over the chicken legs and place them in a dish. Add the fish sauce and soy sauce and turn the chicken to coat well. Cover with plastic wrap and let marinate in the refrigerator for 2 hours.

2   Preheat the broiler to medium-high. Drain the chicken legs, reserving the marinade. Put them on the broiler rack and cook under the preheated broiler, turning and basting frequently with the reserved marinade, for 20–25 minutes, or until the tip of a sharp knife can be inserted into the thickest part of the meat with ease and the juices run clear. A meat thermometer inserted into the thickest part of the meat, without touching the bone, should read 170°F. Garnish with ginger and serve.

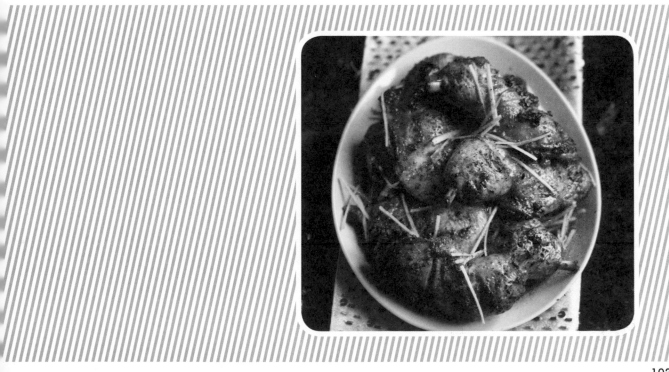

CHICKEN FAJITAS

SERVES 4

3 tablespoons olive oil, plus extra for drizzling

3 tablespoons maple syrup or honey

1 tablespoon red wine vinegar

2 garlic cloves, crushed

2 teaspoons dried oregano

1–2 teaspoons crushed red pepper

4 skinless, boneless chicken breasts

2 red bell peppers, seeded and cut into 1-inch strips

8 tortillas, warmed

salt and pepper, to taste

METHOD

1 Place the oil, maple syrup, vinegar, garlic, oregano, and crushed red pepper in a large, shallow dish or bowl, season with salt and pepper, and mix together.

2 Slice the chicken across the grain into 1-inch-thick slices. Toss in the marinade until well coated. Cover and chill in the refrigerator for 2–3 hours, turning occasionally.

3 Heat a griddle pan or skillet until hot. Lift the chicken slices from the marinade with a slotted spoon, lay on the griddle pan, and cook over medium–high heat for 3–4 minutes on each side, or until cooked through. Remove the chicken to a warm serving plate and keep warm. Add the bell peppers, skin-side down, to the pan and cook for 2 minutes on each side. Transfer to the serving plate. Serve with the warm tortillas to be used as wraps.

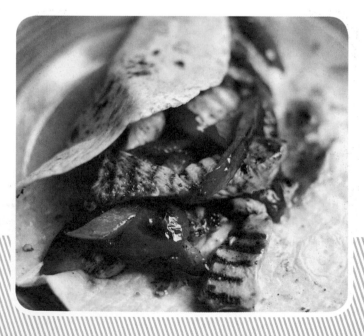

CHICKEN NOODLE SOUP

SERVES 4-6

2 skinless, boneless
chicken breasts

5 cups water or chicken stock

3 carrots, peeled and cut into
½-inch slices

3 ounces vermicelli
(or other small noodles)

salt and pepper, to taste

fresh tarragon leaves,
to garnish

METHOD

1 Place the chicken breasts in a large saucepan, add the water or stock, and bring to a simmer. Cook for 25–30 minutes. Skim any foam from the surface, if necessary. Remove the chicken from the pan and keep warm.

2 Continue to simmer the liquid, add the carrots and vermicelli, and cook for 4–5 minutes, or until the carrots are tender.

3 Thinly slice or shred the chicken breasts and place in warmed serving dishes.

4 Season the soup with salt and pepper to taste and pour over the chicken. Ladle into warmed bowls and serve garnished with the tarragon.

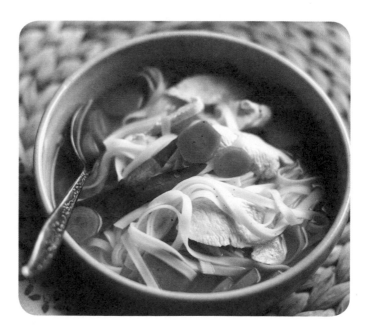

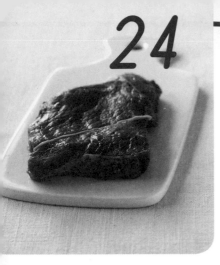

24

GRASS-FED BEEF

Grass-fed beef raised on grazing pasture provides essential fats often lacking in the diet, which can help to keep the skin, bones, and heart healthy.

MAJOR NUTRIENTS PER 3½ OUNCES BEEF, GRASS-FED

Calories	192
Total fat	12.73g
Protein	5.34g
Carbohydrate	19.42g
Fibre	0g
Vitamin B3	4.82mg
Vitamin B5	0.58mg
Vitamin B6	0.36mg
Vitamin 12	1.97mg
Vitamin E	930mg
Iron	1.99mg
Zinc	4.55mg
Selenium	14.2mcg

Grass-fed cattle generally get more exercise, making their meat leaner, and for every 3-ounce serving, there is around ¼ ounce less fat in grass-fed beef than in its grain-fed counterpart. This is good news for calorie-counters, but more importantly, the quality of fat contained in grass-fed beef is better. Grass-fed beef contains high levels of omega-3 oils, which keep the heart, joints, brain, and skin youthful. Another fat, conjugated linoleic acid (CLA), comes direct from the grass, and enables stored fat to be burned as energy, raising the metabolism and helping maintain a trim figure. Low levels of CLA in our diet have been partly linked to the rise of obesity.

• Contains four times more vitamin E than grain-fed beef.
• Good selenium levels lessen anxiety, depression, and fatigue—low levels are associated with heart and bone degeneration.
• Contains the highest level of zinc in any meat, promoting clear skin and strong nails.
• Coenzyme Q-10 increases energy in all cells, especially the heart.

Practical tips:
Ask your butcher for the best source or find a farm shop attached to its own pasture. Top sirloin, tenderloin, and flank steak are the healthiest, leanest cuts. This is a nutrient -dense food, so you need to eat it only 2–4 times a month to get the benefits.

SPICY BEEF STIR-FRY

SERVES 4

1 teaspoon olive oil

5 ounces grass-fed, top sirloin steak, cut into thin strips

1 orange bell pepper, seeded and cut into thin strips

4 scallions, chopped

1–2 fresh jalapeño chiles, seeded and chopped

2–3 garlic cloves, chopped

1½ cups trimmed and diagonally halved snow peas

4 ounces large portobello mushrooms, sliced

1 teaspoon hoisin sauce,

1 tablespoon fresh orange juice

5 cups arugula

METHOD

1 Heat a large wok or skillet over high heat. Add the oil and heat for 30 seconds. Add the beef and stir-fry for 1 minute, or until browned. Using a slotted spoon, remove and reserve.

2 Add the bell pepper, scallions, chiles, and garlic and stir-fry for 2 minutes. Add the snow peas and mushrooms and stir-fry for an additional 2 minutes.

3 Return the beef to the wok and add the hoisin sauce and orange juice. Stir-fry for 2–3 minutes, or until the beef is cooked to your liking and the vegetables are tender but still firm to the bite. Stir in the arugula and stir-fry until it starts to wilt. Serve immediately, divided among four warm bowls.

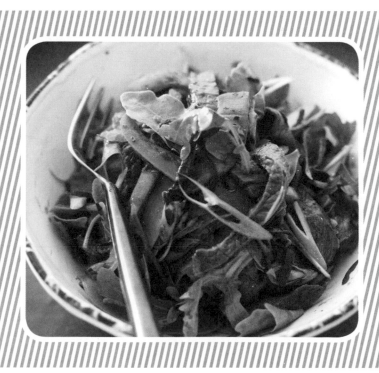

RIB-EYE STEAK IN A BOURBON MARINADE

SERVES 4

4 rib-eye steaks,
12 ounces each
2 tablespoons olive oil
2 tablespoons butter

MARINADE

2 tablespoons extra virgin
olive oil
1 cup good quality bourbon
1 small bunch thyme,
leaves picked
1 teaspoon dried oregano
2 garlic cloves, crushed
1 teaspoon salt
1 teaspoon pepper

METHOD

1   Put all of the marinade ingredients into a shallow, nonmetallic dish that is large enough to hold all of the steaks in a single layer. Mix the ingredients together.

2   Add the steaks to the marinade, turning a few times to coat. Cover and chill in the refrigerator for a minimum of 4 hours, or for up to 12 hours if time allows. Turn once, midway through marinating.

3   Remove from the refrigerator before cooking to let the meat return to room temperature. Reserve the remaining marinade.

4   Preheat a large skillet over high heat and add the oil and butter. Cook the steaks for 5 minutes on each side for medium-rare, or until cooked to your liking. Cook the steaks in batches, if necessary. Set aside to rest for 5 minutes before serving.

5   Meanwhile, reduce the heat to medium-high, pour the reserved marinade into the skillet, and flambé to create a sauce. Serve the steaks with the sauce poured over the top.

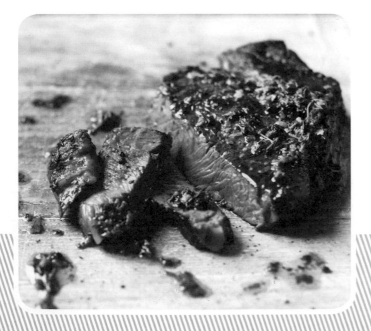

BEEF CHILI

SERVES 6

2 tablespoons olive oil
1 onion, chopped
1 red bell pepper, diced
3 garlic cloves, minced
1 pound fresh ground beef
2 tablespoons chili powder
½ teaspoon cayenne pepper
1 (14½-ounce) can diced
tomatoes
1¾ cups water
2 tablespoons chopped
fresh parsley
salt and pepper, to taste

METHOD

1. Heat 1 tablespoon of the oil in a large, heavy saucepan over medium heat. Add the onion, red bell pepper, and garlic and sauté for about 5 minutes, stirring, until tender. Remove the sautéed vegetables from the pan, then add the remaining oil.

2. When hot, add the ground beef with the chili powder and cayenne pepper, and season with salt and pepper. Stir to coat the meat with the spices and sauté for about 10 minutes, stirring frequently and breaking up the meat with a wooden spoon, until brown.

3. Add the sautéed vegetables, the tomatoes with their can juices, and the water to the pan. Bring to a boil, reduce the heat, and simmer for about 45 minutes, stirring occasionally, until the sauce is thick. Season with salt and pepper and stir in the parsley.

4. Serve immediately or let cool and store in the refrigerator, covered, for up to 4 days before using.

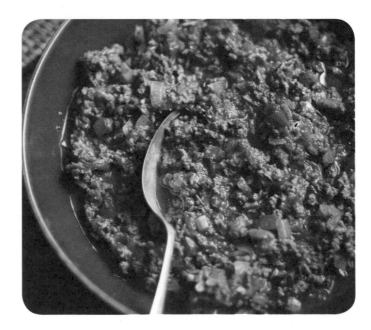

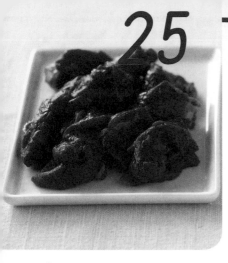

25

VENISON

Venison has recently grown in popularity. It is similar to beef but is leaner, providing dense protein without the heart-clogging saturated-fat content.

MAJOR NUTRIENTS PER 3½ OUNCES VENISON

Calories	157
Total fat	7.13g
Saturadted fat	3.36g
Protein	21.78g
Carbohydrate	0mg
Fibre	0mg
Vitamin B2	0.55mg
Vitamin B3	0.69mg
Vitamin B5	0.75mg
Vitamin B6	32mcg
Vitamin B12	3.15g
Iron	2.92g
Zinc	4.2mg
Selenium	10mg

This protein combines with a great B-vitamin profile to keep the body intact and youthful. It includes the sulfur-containing amino acids taurine and cystine, which are key in aiding the liver to rid the body of toxins as part of the metabolic process. If these are allowed to keep circulating, the body becomes tired, ill, and unable to heal and renew. Taurine and cystine also help hold essential minerals in the body, tone the blood, prevent heart disease, and improve circulation to keep skin healthy and glowing.

• Vitamins B12 and B6 clear the brain and heart of the substance homocysteine, which can lead to dementia and heart disease.
• Vitamin B3 keeps joints mobile and prevents osteoarthritis.
• Contains zinc, which revitalizes the skin and keeps pores clear.
• Zinc and selenium in combination create detoxification enzymes that rejuvenate cells all over the body.
• Iron moves oxygen around the body for efficient healing.

Practical tips:
Ask your butcher to let you know when venison is in season. If you buy at this time, from animals that have been hunted, you'll benefit from an absence of aging additives. Venison should be frozen for a minimum of two hours before use to kill off any parasites or tapeworms. Broil venison steaks and cook less tender cuts in a hearty winter stew with root vegetables and spices.

CHARBROILED VENISON STEAKS

SERVES 4

4 venison steaks
fresh thyme sprigs, to garnish

MARINADE
⅔ cup red wine
2 tablespoons olive oil
1 tablespoon red wine vinegar
1 onion, chopped
1 tablespoon chopped fresh parsley
1 tablespoon chopped fresh thyme
1 bay leaf
1 teaspoon good-quality honey
½ teaspoon mild mustard
salt and pepper

METHOD

1 Place the venison steaks in a shallow, nonmetallic dish.

2 To make the marinade, add the wine, oil, wine vinegar, onion, fresh parsley, thyme, bay leaf, honey, and mustard to a bowl, season with salt and pepper, and beat vigorously, until well combined.

3 Pour the marinade over the venison, cover, and let marinate in the refrigerator overnight. Turn the steaks occasionally so that the meat is well coated.

4 Preheat the broiler to high. Cook the venison under the hot broiler for 2 minutes on each side to seal the meat.

5 Turn down the broiler to medium, and cook for an additional 4–10 minutes on each side, according to taste. Test by inserting the tip of a knife into the meat—the juices will range from red when the meat is still rare to clear as the meat becomes well cooked.

6 Transfer the steaks to serving plates, garnish with fresh thyme sprigs, and serve.

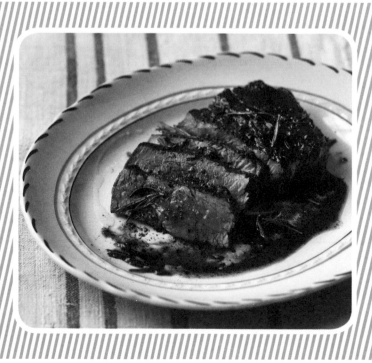

VENISON CASSEROLE

SERVES 6

3 tablespoons olive oil

2 pound 4 ounces casserole venison, cut into 1¼-inch cubes

2 onions, finely sliced

2 garlic cloves, chopped

1½ cups beef stock or vegetable stock

2 tablespoons all-purpose flour

½ cup port or red wine

2 tablespoons red currant jelly

6 juniper berries, crushed

4 cloves, crushed

pinch of cinnamon

small grating of nutmeg

salt and pepper, to taste

mashed potatoes, to serve

METHOD

1 Preheat the oven to 350°F. Heat the oil in a large, flameproof casserole and cook the venison over high heat, stirring frequently, for 5 minutes, or until browned on all sides and sealed. Transfer to a large plate using a slotted spoon.

2 Add the onion and garlic to the casserole and cook over medium heat, stirring frequently, for 5 minutes, or until softened. Transfer to the plate with the meat.

3 Gradually stir in the stock and scrape any sediment from the bottom of the casserole, then bring to a boil, stirring.

4 Sprinkle the flour over the meat, onions, and garlic on the plate, and toss well to coat evenly. Return to the casserole and stir well, making sure that the meat is just covered with the stock. Stir in the port or wine, red currant jelly, and spices.

5 Season well with salt and pepper, then cover and cook in the center of the preheated oven for 2–2½ hours.

6 Check and adjust the seasoning if necessary, then serve with mashed potatoes.

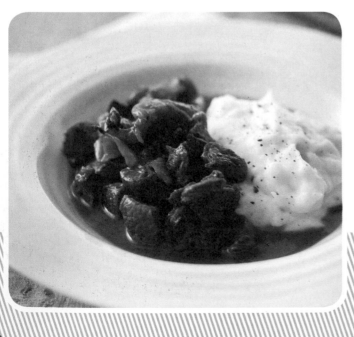

VENISON & MUSHROOM PIE

SERVES 4-6

2 pounds casserole venison,
cut into 1-inch cubes
4 tablespoons all-purpose
flour
1 teaspoon dried thyme
1 stick butter
2 onions, thinly sliced
2 carrots, thinly sliced
5 ounces mushrooms, sliced
2¼ cups beef stock
1¾ cups brown ale, or stout
15 ounces store-bought
puff pastry
1 egg, beaten
salt and pepper, to taste

METHOD

1   Mix together the venison, flour, and thyme, and season
generously with salt and pepper. Melt the butter in a large pan,
add the venison and cook over medium heat for 10 minutes,
until browned. Add the onions, carrots, and mushrooms, pour in
the stock and ale, and bring to a boil.

2   Reduce the heat, cover and simmer for 1½–2 hours, stirring
occasionally. Transfer the mixture to a large pie dish and leave
to cool.

3   Preheat the oven to 400°F.

4   Roll out the pastry on a floured surface to 1 inch larger than
the top of the dish. Cut out a ½-inch strip all the way around.
Brush the rim of the dish with water and press the strip on it.
Brush with water and lift the remaining dough on top. Trim off
the excess and crimp the edges to seal. Make a small slit in the
center and brush with beaten egg. Roll out the trimmings and
use to decorate the pie, then brush all over with beaten egg.
Bake for 35–40 minutes, until golden brown. Serve immediately.

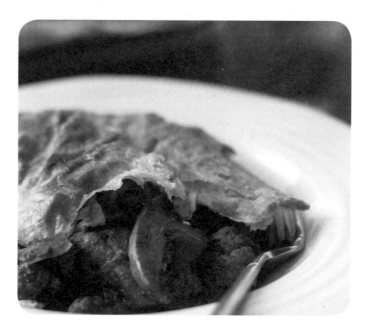

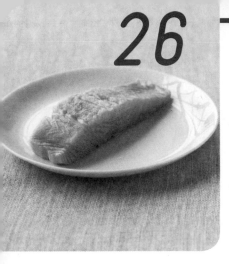

26

SALMON

Salmon is an excellent source of omega-3 fats, cancer-fighting selenium, and vitamin B12, which helps protect against heart disease and a form of anemia.

MAJOR NUTRIENTS PER 3½ OUNCES SALMON

Calories	183
Total fat	10.8g
Protein	19.9g
EPA	0.618g
DHA	1.293g
Niacin	7.5mg
Vitamin B6	0.64mcg
Vitamin B12	2573mcg
Folate	123mcg
Vitamin E	1.9mg
Vitamin C	3.9mg
Potassium	362mcg
Selenium	36.5mcg
Magnesium	28mg
Zinc	0.4mg

The salmon that we eat today is often farmed instead of wild. Although wild salmon tends to contain less fat and slightly higher levels of some nutrients, the two kinds are broadly comparable. Salmon is an important source of fish oils, which provide protection against heart disease, blood clots, strokes, high blood pressure, high blood cholesterol, Alzheimer's disease, depression, and certain skin conditions. Salmon is also an excellent source of selenium, which protects against cancer, plus protein, niacin, vitamin B12, magnesium, and vitamin B6.

• Protection against cardiovascular diseases and strokes.
• Helps keep the brain healthy and improve insulin resistance.
• Contains good levels of docosahexaenoic (DHA) and eicosapentaenoic acid (EPA)—vital for maintaining brain and eye health.
• Helps minimize joint pain and may protect against cancers.

Practical tips:
Where possible, buy wild salmon—although just as high in nutrients, farmed salmon has been found to contain up to twice the amount of fat. For optimum omega-3 content, instead of pan-frying, cook salmon lightly and poach or broil. Overcooking can oxidize the essential fats, and this means that they are no longer beneficial. Frozen salmon retains the beneficial oils, vitamins, and minerals, while canned salmon loses a proportion of these nutrients.

BROILED SALMON WITH CITRUS SALSA

SERVES 4

4 salmon fillets
1 tablespoon olive oil
1 tablespoon light soy sauce
salt and pepper, to taste

CITRUS SALSA

1 large orange
1 lime
2 tomatoes, peeled and diced
2 tablespoons extra virgin olive oil
2 tablespoons chopped fresh cilantro
¼ teaspoon granulated sugar

METHOD

1 Preheat the broiler to high. To make the salsa, cut all the peel and white pith from the orange and lime and remove the segments, discarding the membranes and reserving the juices.

2 Chop the segments and mix with the reserved juice, the tomatoes, oil, and cilantro. Add the sugar and season with salt and pepper.

3 Place the salmon fillets on the broiler rack. Mix together the oil and soy sauce, brush over the salmon, and season with pepper. Place under the preheated broiler and cook, turning once, for 8–10 minutes, until the fish is firm and flakes easily.

4 Serve the salmon with a spoonful of citrus salsa on the side.

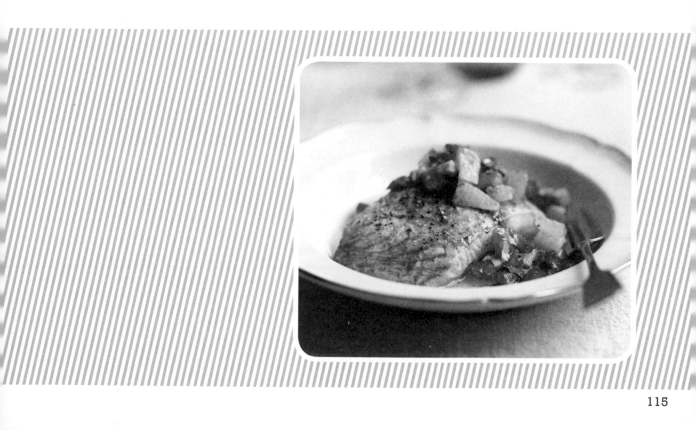

MINI SALMON & BROCCOLI PIES

MAKES ABOUT 8

2 cups broccoli florets
4 ounce cooked salmon fillet
15 ounces rolled pie crust dough
flour, for dusting
1 egg, beaten
salad, to serve
salt and pepper, to taste

WHITE SAUCE

2 tablespoons butter
¼ cup all-purpose flour
1¼ cups warm milk

METHOD

1 Cook the broccoli in lightly salted boiling water for 5–10 minutes, until tender. Drain and let cool.

2 To make the white sauce, melt the butter in a saucepan, add the flour, and cook over low heat, stirring continuously, for 2 minutes. Gradually stir in the warm milk. Bring to a boil, stirring continuously, then simmer, stirring, until thickened and smooth. Season, remove from the heat, and let cool, stirring occasionally.

3 Flake the flesh of the salmon into a bowl. Break up the broccoli florets and add to the bowl. Stir in the white sauce and season with salt and pepper. Mix well.

4 Preheat the oven to 400°F. Roll out the dough on a lightly floured surface and stamp out 16 circles with a 4-inch cutter. Put 8 circles into a muffin pan. Add spoonfuls of the salmon mixture without filling the pastry shells completely. Brush the edges of the remaining circles with water and use to cover the pies, pressing with the tines of a fork to seal.

5 Brush the tops with the beaten egg and bake for 20–25 minutes, until golden brown. Serve with salad.

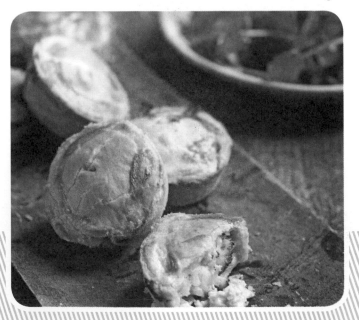

SMOKED SALMON RISOTTO

SERVES 4

4 tablespoons unsalted butter

1 onion, finely chopped

½ small fennel bulb, finely chopped

2½ cups risotto rice

1¼ cups white wine or vermouth

5 cups hot fish stock

6 ounces hot smoked salmon, flaked

6 ounces smoked salmon slices

2 tablespoons fresh chervil leaves or chopped flat-leaf parsley

salt and pepper, to taste

METHOD

1 Melt half the butter in a large saucepan over medium heat, add the onion and fennel, and cook, stirring frequently, for 5–8 minutes, until transparent and soft. Add the rice and stir well to coat the grains in the butter. Cook, stirring, for 3 minutes, then add the wine, stir, and let simmer until most of the liquid has been absorbed.

2 With the stock simmering in a separate saucepan, add a ladleful to the rice and stir well. Cook, stirring continuously, until nearly all the liquid has been absorbed before adding another ladleful of stock. Continue to add the remaining stock in the same way until the rice is cooked but still firm to the bite and most or all of the stock has been added.

3 Remove from the heat and stir in the two types of salmon and the remaining butter. Season with salt and pepper and serve sprinkled with the chervil.

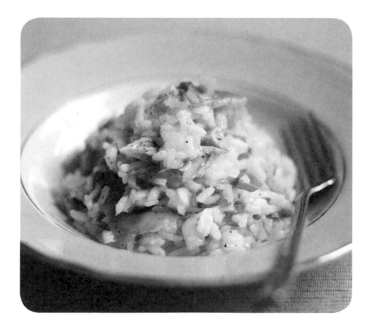

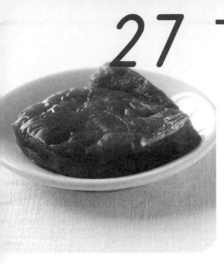

27

TUNA

Fresh tuna is an important source of omega-3 fats and antioxidant minerals for arterial and heart health, and it is also rich in vitamin E for healthy skin.

MAJOR NUTRIENTS PER 3½ OUNCES TUNA

Calories	144
Total fat	4.9g
Protein	23g
EPA	0.4g
DHA	1.2g
Niacin	8.3mg
Vitamin B5	1mg
Vitamin B6	0.5mg
Vitamin B12	9.4mg
Vitamin E	1mg
Potassium	252mg
Selenium	36mcg
Magnesium	50mg
Iron	1mg
Zinc	0.6mg

DID YOU KNOW?

Research has found that when tuna is canned it loses most of its beneficial omega-3 fats, so it shouldn't count toward your oily fish intake.

The firm, meaty flesh of fresh or frozen tuna is an ideal choice of fish for non-fish-lovers and is also simple to prepare and quick to cook. It is an excellent source of protein and is especially rich in the B vitamins, selenium, and magnesium. A small portion will contain around 20 percent of your daily vitamin E needs. While most types of tuna contain fewer of the essential omega-3 fats than some other oily fishes, there is still a good content of benefical fats. DHA fats are particularly effective in keeping our hearts and brains healthy and in good working order. Just one portion of tuna a week can provide the recommended 1.4 g of these fats a week.

• A good source of omega-3, EPA, and DHA fats, which offer protection against a range of diseases.
• Rich in selenium and magnesium for heart health.
• Extremely rich in vitamin B12 for healthy blood.

Practical tips:
Fresh fish should be odorless, with bright, clear eyes, and it is best cooked and eaten on the day of purchase. To retain all the health benefits of the omega-3 fats, lightly sear tuna in a skillet on both sides and cook for as little time as you can. Tuna steaks can also be sliced and stir-fried with vegetables—unlike many types of fish, it has a meaty texture and the slices won't disintegrate when cooked.

TUNA & TOMATO PITA POCKETS

SERVES 4

4 pita breads

1 butterhead lettuce, coarsely shredded

8 cherry tomatoes, halved

1 (12-ounce) can tuna in oil, drained and flaked

½ cup mayonnaise

1 teaspoon finely grated lemon rind

2 tablespoons lemon juice

3 tablespoons chopped fresh chives

salt and pepper, to taste

METHOD

1 Cut the pita breads in half and open them out to make a pocket.

2 Divide the lettuce among the pitas, then add the tomatoes and tuna.

3 Put the mayonnaise, lemon rind, lemon juice, and chives into a bowl and mix together. Season with salt and pepper and spoon over the pita filling to serve.

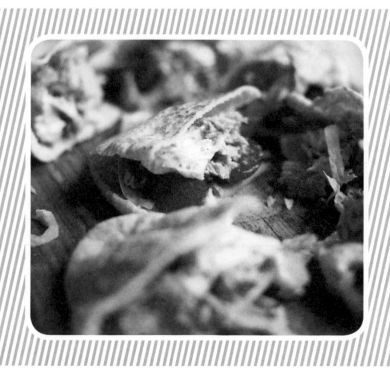

TUNA STEAKS WITH FRUITY SALSA

SERVES 2

2 tuna steaks, about
5 ounces each

olive oil, for brushing

salt and pepper, to taste

mixed salad leaves,
to serve

FRUITY SALSA

1 mango, diced

¼ red onion, diced

1-inch cucumber slice, diced

½ firm tomato, diced

½ tablespoon chopped
pickled jalapeño

1½ tablespoons chopped
fresh coriander

juice and zest of ½ lime

METHOD

1 To make the salsa, mix the mango, red onion, cucumber, tomato, jalapeño and coriander with the juice and zest of the lime. Stir well and set aside for 15 minutes to let the flavors develop.

2 Preheat a griddle pan until very hot. Brush both sides of the tuna steaks lightly with oil then season with salt and pepper. Cook on the hot pan for 2 minutes on each side, or until seared on the outside and rare in the middle, or according to personal taste.

3 Transfer the tuna steaks to serving plates and spoon the salsa over the top. Serve immediately, with mixed salad leaves on the side.

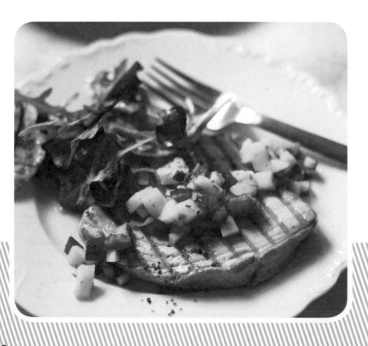

TUNA SASHIMI

SERVES 4

2 carrots, grated

1 celery stalk, thinly sliced

1 small red onion, thinly sliced

1-inch piece fresh ginger, grated

12 ounces fresh tuna fillet

1 teaspoon sesame seeds, to serve

DRESSING

3 tablespoons rice vinegar or white wine vinegar

1 tablespoon lemon juice

2 tablespoons shoyu or soy sauce

1 teaspoon sesame oil

METHOD

1. To make the dressing, put the vinegar, lemon juice, shoyu, and sesame oil in a jar and shake well to mix.

2. Put the carrots, celery, onion, and ginger in a bowl and stir to mix. Pour over half of the dressing and toss to coat evenly.

3. Arrange the salad on four serving plates. Using a sharp knife, slice the tuna thinly and arrange the slices over the salad.

4. Spoon the remaining dressing over the tuna and serve sprinkled with sesame seeds.

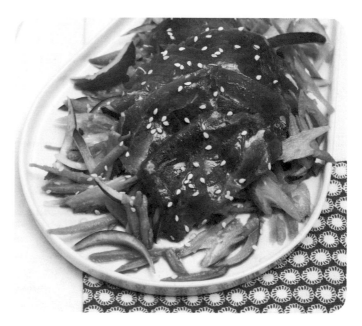

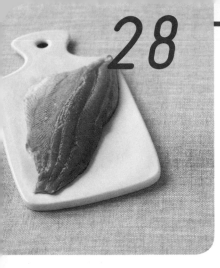

28

TROUT

Trout is one of a number of oily fish sources that provide a valuable package of nutrients that safeguard the joints, eyes, and brain from damage.

MAJOR NUTRIENTS PER 3½ OUNCES SMOKED TROUT

Calories	148
Total fat	6.61g
EPA	0.2g
DHA	0.53g
Protein	20.77g
Carbohydrate	0mg
Fibre	0mg
Vitamin B1	0.35mg
Vitamin B3	4.5mg
Vitamin B12	7.79mg
Vitamin D	155 IU

Omega-3 oils are crucial to mood and behavior regulation because they affect how we use the stabilizing brain chemicals serotonin and dopamine. Eating oily fish one to three times a week has also been shown to improve brain function and slow down the loss in concentration, memory, and mental acuity associated with aging and stress. Of all the oily fish, trout is one of the least contaminated by mercury toxicity. Mercury is common in larger oily fish, such as tuna and swordfish, and, therefore, it should be avoided by young children and pregnant women.

- Contains pink astaxanthin, which supports good eye health and brain development.
- Contains vitamin D—low levels of which have been linked to occurrences of both depression and dementia.
- High levels of the B vitamins promote increased energy levels.
- Omega-3 oils lubricate joints to aid pain-free agility.

Practical tips:
Trout can be bought both fresh and smoked. The fresh fish are easy to stuff with herbs and lemon and bake, and the smoked type makes a good alternative to the stronger-flavored salmon. This is an excellent choice of oily fish for people who dislike a strong fishy flavor.

SMOKED TROUT SALAD

SERVES 4

1 red bell pepper, halved and seeded

4 smoked trout fillets, about 5 ounces each, skinned and flaked

4 scallions, trimmed and chopped

2 large chicory heads, halved, cored, and shredded

1½ tablespoons Chinese rice wine vinegar

½ tablespoon sunflower oil

2 tablespoons chopped fresh parsley

radicchio leaves, rinsed and dried

salt and pepper, to taste

METHOD

1 Run a swivel-bladed vegetable peeler along the length of the cut edges of the bell pepper to make very thin slices. Chop the slices and put them in a bowl.

2 Add the trout, scallions, and chicory, tossing to mix together. Add 1 tablespoon of the vinegar, the oil, parsley, and salt and pepper and toss again, then add extra vinegar as required.

3 Cover and chill until ready to serve. Arrange the radicchio leaves on individual plates. Toss the salad again and adjust the seasoning, if necessary. Place a portion of salad on each plate of radicchio leaves and serve.

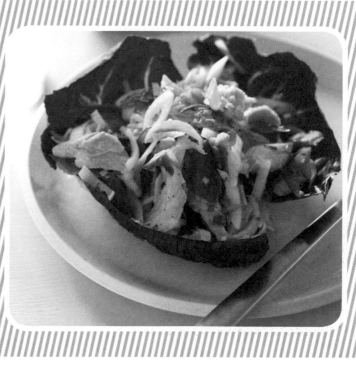

PENANG FISH CURRY

SERVES 4

4 tablespoons peanuts, toasted
8–10 shallots, chopped
2–3 fresh red chiles, chopped
1-inch piece fresh ginger,
chopped
4 large garlic cloves, chopped
1 teaspoon shrimp paste
4 tablespoons peanut oil
1 teaspoon ground turmeric
½ teaspoon chili powder
scant 2 cups lukewarm water
½ teaspoon salt, or to taste
2 tablespoons tamarind juice
½ teaspoon sugar
1 pound 9 ounces skinless
trout fillets, cut into
½-inch slices
fresh cilantro sprigs,
to garnish

METHOD

1   Put the peanuts, shallots, chiles, ginger, garlic, and shrimp paste in a food processor or blender and process until the mixture forms a rough paste. Remove and set aside.

2   Heat a large, shallow saucepan over medium heat, then add the oil. Add the peanut mixture, turmeric, and chili powder. Cook, stirring frequently, until the mixture begins to brown, then continue to cook for 10–12 minutes, until the mixture is fragrant, occasionally adding a little water to prevent the mixture from sticking to the bottom of the pan.

3   Pour in the lukewarm water and add the salt, tamarind juice, and sugar. Stir and mix well and carefully add the fish. Stir gently to make sure that the fish is covered with the sauce. Cover the pan, reduce the heat to low, and cook for 8–10 minutes. Remove from the heat and serve immediately, garnished with cilantro sprigs and accompanied by rice.

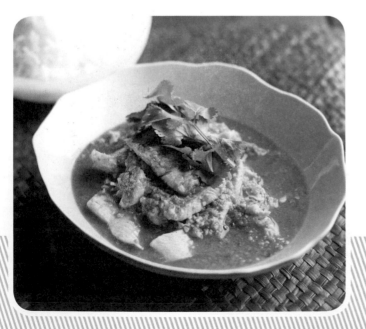

TROUT WITH WATERCRESS SAUCE

SERVES 4

4 whole trout, about 12 ounces each, cleaned

olive oil, for greasing

1 small bunch fresh flat-leaf parsley

1 small bunch fresh chives

1 lemon, thinly sliced

salt and pepper

lemon wedges, to serve

WATERCRESS SAUCE

2 bunches watercress, coarse stalks discarded, coarsely chopped

juice of ½ lemon

3 tablespoons vegetable or fish stock

¼ teaspoon salt

¼ teaspoon pepper

4 tablespoons heavy cream

4 tablespoons plain yogurt

METHOD

1 Preheat the barbecue. Remove the heads from the trout and make 2 diagonal slashes on each side in the thickest part of the flesh, about 3½ inches apart. Brush all over with oil. Stuff the slashes and the body cavity with parsley, chives, and lemon slices. Season to taste with salt and pepper. Grease a hinged wire basket and place the trout in it.

2 For the sauce, put the watercress, lemon juice, stock, salt, and pepper in a food processor. Blend for 2–3 minutes, scraping down the sides of the bowl frequently. Pour into a pitcher, stir in the cream and yogurt, and mix well.

3 Grease the grill rack. Cook the trout over hot coals for 5–6 minutes each side, or until cooked through. Carefully remove the trout from the basket, using the tip of a knife to ease the skin away from the wire. Serve on warmed plates with lemon wedges and the watercress sauce.

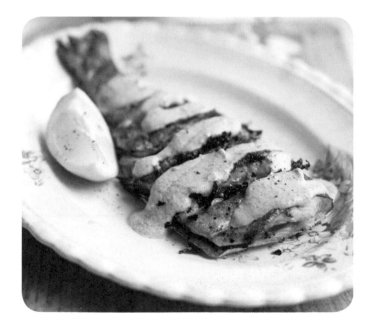

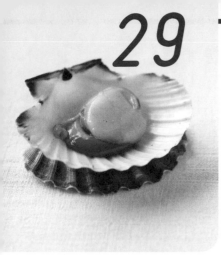

29

SCALLOPS

They may be a luxurious treat but scallops can also help boost your vitamin B12 and magnesium intake, which, in turn, could help to protect the arteries and bones.

Scallops are an excellent source of vitamin B12, which is needed by the body to deactivate homocysteine, a chemical that can damage blood-vessel walls. High homocysteine levels are also linked to osteoporosis. A recent study found that osteoporosis occurred more frequently among women whose vitamin B12 was deficient. B12 is particularly important for individuals who don't consume red meat as a regular part of their diet. Scallops are also a good source of magnesium and a regular intake helps build bone density, regulate nerves, and keep the heart healthy.

- Low in calories and fat so ideal for dieters.
- Rich in magnesium, which is essential to all cells—magnesium deficiency has been linked to illnesses, such as asthma, diabetes, and osteoporosis.
- A good source of vitamin B12 for arterial and bone health.
- Regular intake may help protect against colon cancer.

Practical tips:
Fresh scallops should have flesh that is white and firm, have no evidence of browning, and be free of odor. The orange-pink coral can be either removed or cooked along with the rest of the scallop. Scallops should be cooked for only a few minutes, because exposure to too much heat will cause them to become tough. The sweet flavor of scallops goes well with chile, cilantro, garlic, and parsley.

MAJOR NUTRIENTS PER 3½ OUNCES SHELLED SCALLOPS

Calories	88
Total fat	0.8g
Protein	16.8g
Vitamin B12	1.5g
Folate	16mcg
Potassium	314mg
Selenium	22mcg
Magnesium	56mg
Zinc	0.95mg
Calsium	24mg

DID YOU KNOW?

Scallops are rich in tryptophan, an amino acid that helps the production of the mood-enhancing serotonin in our brains and may help cure insomnia.

SPICY SCALLOPS WITH LIME & CHILE

SERVES 4

16 large scallops, shelled
1 tbsp butter
1 tablespoon vegetable oil
1 teaspoon crushed garlic
1 teaspoon grated fresh ginger
1 bunch of scallions, finely sliced
finely grated rind of 1 lime
1 small fresh red chile, seeded and very finely chopped
3 tablespoons lime juice
lime wedges, to garnish
freshly cooked rice, to serve

METHOD

1 Using a sharp knife, trim the scallops to remove the dark vein, then wash and pat dry with paper towels. Separate the corals from the white parts and discard, then slice the remaining scallops in half horizontally, making 2 circles from each.

2 Heat the butter and oil in a preheated wok. Add the garlic and ginger and stir-fry for 1 minute without browning. Add the scallions and stir-fry for 1 minute.

3 Add the scallops and continue stir-frying over high heat for 4–5 minutes. Stir in the lime rind, chile, and lime juice and cook for an additional 1 minute.

4 Transfer the scallops to serving plates, then spoon over the cooking juices and garnish with lime wedges. Serve hot with freshly cooked rice.

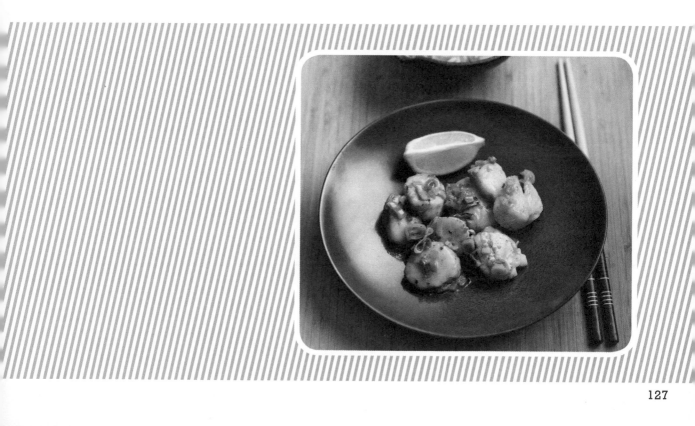

SCALLOPS WITH BREAD CRUMBS

SERVES 4

20 large fresh scallops, removed from their shells

1¾ sticks salted butter, plus extra, if needed

3 slices day-old bread, made into fine bread crumbs

4 garlic cloves, finely chopped

⅓ cup finely chopped fresh flat-leaf parsley

salt and pepper, to taste

lemon wedges, to serve

METHOD

1 Preheat the oven to 225°F. Use a small knife to remove the dark vein that runs around each scallop, then rinse and pat dry. Season with salt and pepper and set aside.

2 Melt half of the butter in a large sauté pan or skillet over high heat. Add the bread crumbs and garlic, reduce the heat to medium, and sauté, stirring, for 5–6 minutes, or until golden brown. Remove the garlic bread crumbs from the pan and drain well on paper towels, then keep warm in the oven. Wipe out the pan.

3 Use two large sauté pans or skillets to cook all the scallops at once without overcrowding the pans. Melt 3½ tablespoons of the remaining butter in each pan over high heat. Reduce the heat to medium, divide the scallops between the two pans and cook for 2 minutes.

4 Turn the scallops over and continue cooking for an additional 2–3 minutes, or until they are golden and cooked through. Add extra butter to the pans, if necessary.

5 Sprinkle with the bread crumbs and parsley, and serve with lemon wedges for squeezing over.

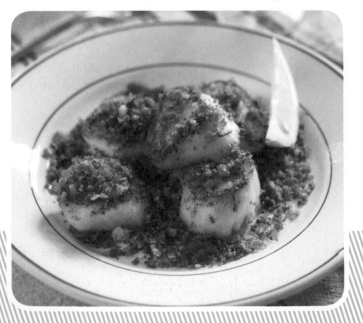

SCALLOPS IN BLACK BEAN SAUCE

SERVES 4

2 tablespoons vegetable oil

1 teaspoon finely chopped garlic

1 teaspoon finely chopped fresh ginger

1 tablespoon fermented black beans, rinsed and lightly mashed

14 ounces prepared scallops

½ teaspoon light soy sauce

1 teaspoon Chinese rice wine

1 teaspoon sugar

3–4 fresh red Thai chiles, finely chopped

1–2 teaspoon chicken stock

1 tablespoon finely chopped scallions

METHOD

1   Heat a wok over medium–high heat and add the oil. Add the garlic and stir, then add the ginger and stir fry together for about 1 minute, until fragrant. Mix in the black beans, add the scallops and stir-fry for 1 minute. Add the light soy sauce, rice wine, sugar, and chiles.

2   Lower the heat and simmer for 2 minutes or until the scallops are cooked through. Then add the stock. Finally, add the scallions, stir and serve.

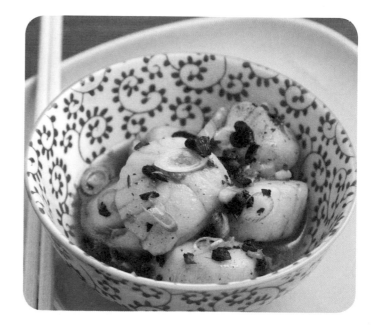

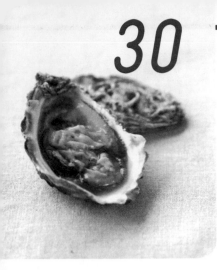

30

OYSTERS

Rich in zinc, oysters are prized for their nutritional qualities, which are thought to boost the immune system and aid the body's healing process.

Although there is little scientific evidence that oysters are an aphrodisiac, they are one of our best sources of zinc—and this mineral is strongly linked with fertility and virility. Zinc is also important for skin health and the immune system, and it is an antioxidant. Recent research has found that ceramide compounds in oysters inhibit the growth of breast cancer cells. Oysters also contain reasonable amounts of essential omega-3 fats, are rich in selenium for a healthy immune system, and contain easily absorbed iron for energy and healthy blood.

- Excellent source of zinc for fertility and virility.
- Contain compounds and materials that can protect against cancers.
- High iron content for energy, resistance to infection, and healthy blood.
- A good source of the B vitamins.

Practical tips:
Oysters need to be very fresh and, if eaten raw, they should be alive. It is safest to eat farmed oysters because, in recent years, wild oysters have been found to contain toxic levels of contaminants. To prepare fresh oysters, scrub the shells with a stiff brush under cold water. Discard any that are cracked or damaged, or whose shells do not snap shut when tapped—this means that the oyster inside is dead.

MAJOR NUTRIENTS PER 6 OYSTERS

Calories	50
Total fat	1.3g
Protein	4.4g
Vitamin B12	3.9g
Folate	15g
Selenium	53.5mg
Magnesium	28mg
Zinc	31.8mg
Calcium	37mg
Iron	4.9mcg

DID YOU KNOW?

Traditionally, an oyster is eaten in one swallow from the shell, without chewing. You can also cook oysters, but some of the beneficial compounds may be lost.

OYSTERS ROCKEFELLER

SERVES 4

24 fresh oysters

kosher salt

1 tablespoon unsalted butter

2 tablespoons light olive oil

6 scallions, chopped

1 large garlic clove, crushed

3 tablespoons finely chopped celery

15 watercress sprigs

3 cups young spinach leaves, rinsed and trimmed

1 tablespoon anise-flavored liqueur

¼ cup fresh bread crumbs

few drops of hot pepper sauce, to taste

¼ teaspoon pepper

lemon wedges, to serve

METHOD

1 Preheat the oven to 400°F. Shuck the oysters, running an oyster knife under each oyster to loosen it from its shell. Pour off the liquid. Arrange a ½-inch layer of salt in a roasting pan large enough to hold the oysters in a single layer. Nestle the oyster shells in the salt so that they remain upright. Cover with a damp dish towel and chill while you prepare the topping.

2 Melt half the butter and the oil in a large skillet. Add the scallions, garlic, and celery and cook over medium heat, stirring frequently, for 2–3 minutes, or until softened.

3 Stir in the remaining butter, then add the watercress and spinach and cook for 1 minute, or until the leaves wilt. Transfer to a small food processor or blender and add the remaining ingredients. Process until well blended.

4 Spoon 2–3 teaspoons of the sauce over each oyster. Bake in the preheated oven for 20 minutes. Serve with lemon wedges for squeezing over the scallops.

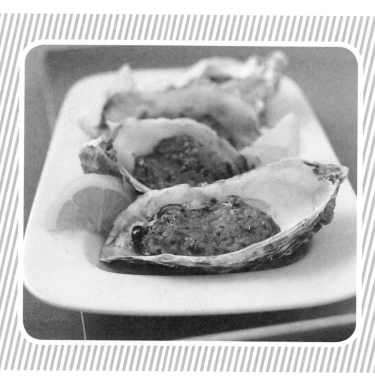

OYSTERS WITH PANCETTA-SHALLOT BUTTER

SERVES 4

12 fresh oysters in the shell

PANCETTA-SHALLOT BUTTER
2 ounces pancetta, chopped
1 shallot, chopped
1 stick unsalted butter
1 tablespoon chopped fresh
flat-leaf parsley
salt

METHOD

1   To make the butter, heat a skillet on the stove over medium–
    high heat. Add the pancetta and shallot and cook for about
    5 minutes, stirring, until the shallot is soft and translucent and
    the pancetta is beginning to get crisp. Remove from the heat
    and let cool.

2   Combine the butter, pancetta–shallot mixture (discarding any
    rendered fat in the skillet), and parsley. Stir to mix and add salt
    to taste.

3   Preheat the broiler to high. Scrub the oysters with a stiff brush
    and rinse under cold running water. Discard any open oysters
    that don't close when you wash them.

4   Place the oysters under the preheated broiler, rounded side
    up. Broil for about 10 minutes, until the shells pop open and the
    juice bubbles out. Remove from the heat and pry off the flat side
    of the shells, retaining the juice and meat in the bottom shells.
    Sever the muscle that attaches the oyster to the shell.
    As each oyster is prepared, spoon some of the butter on top.
    Serve immediately.

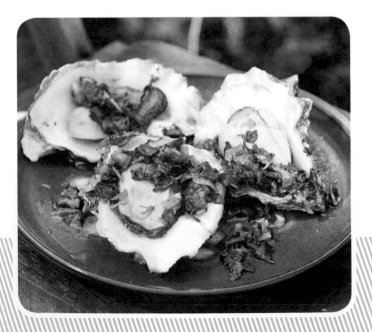

OYSTERS VALENTINO

SERVES 2

12 fresh oysters

4 tablespoons fresh bread crumbs

2 tablespoons diced red pepper

1 tablespoon finely chopped scallions

1 tablespoon chopped fresh parsley

zest of 1 lime

hot pepper sauce, plus extra to serve (optional)

3 tablespoons freshly grated Parmesan cheese

METHOD

1. To open the oysters, hold them flat-side up, above a sieve set over a bowl to catch the juices. Insert the point of an oyster knife into the hinge and work it around until you can prise off the top shell and discard. Loosen the oyster from the deep shell and strain off and reserve the juice.

2. Crumple a sheet of foil and place in a broiler pan. Arrange the shells in the pan using the foil to help them sit flat. Preheat the broiler to high.

3. In a small bowl, mix the bread crumbs, red pepper, scallions, parsley, and lime zest. Add enough of the oyster juice to moisten and a few drops of hot pepper sauce, if liked, and divide the mixture among the oysters.

4. Sprinkle each one with a little Parmesan cheese and cook under the preheated broiler for 3–4 minutes, or until golden and bubbling. Serve immediately with more hot pepper sauce, if liked.

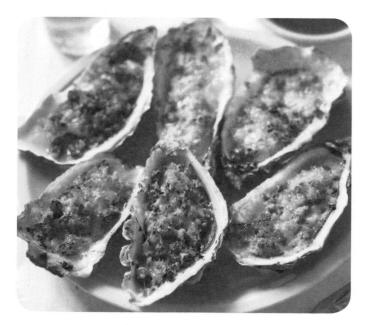

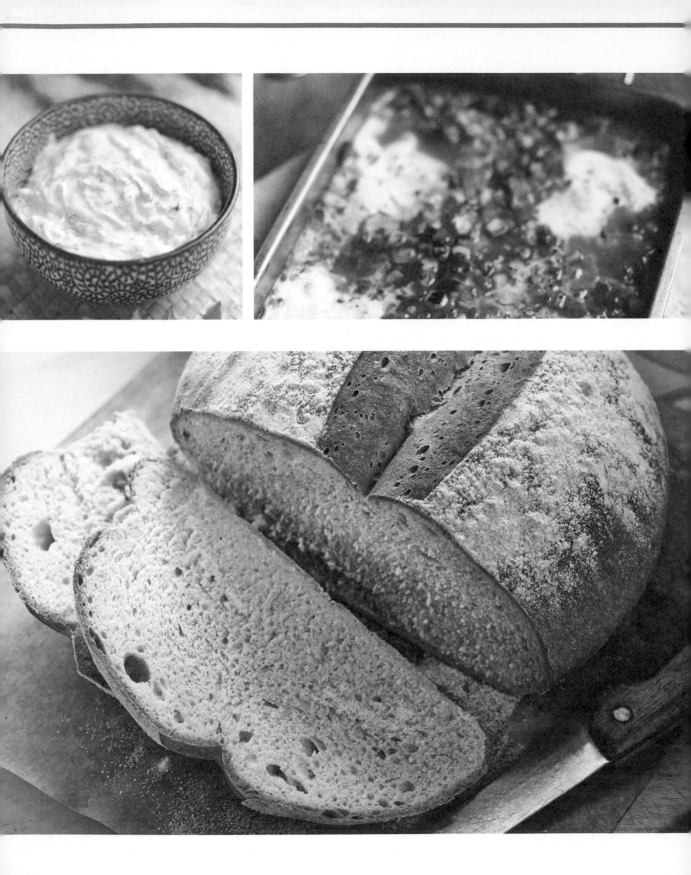

DAIRY & EGGS

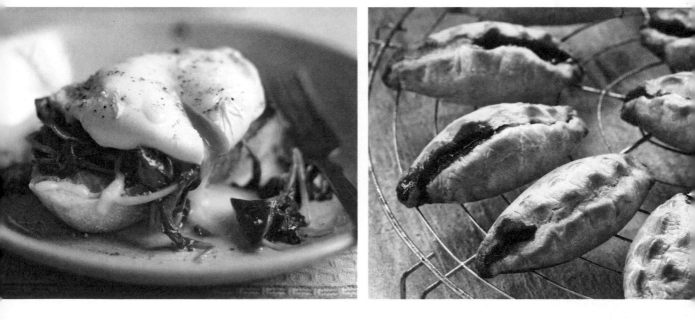

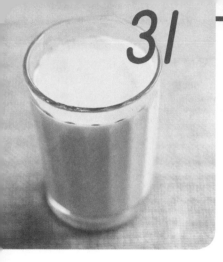

31

KEFIR

Although kefir is less well known than its cousin yogurt, its rejuvenating, immune-enhancing properties are making it increasingly popular.

MAJOR NUTRIENTS PER ½ CUP KEFIR

Calories	61
Total fat	Varies
Protein	Varies
Carbohydrate	Varies
Calcium	1.2g
Potassium	120mg
Zinc	0.36mg

Adding kefir to the diet provides an extra dimension to the immune-supporting actions of fermented foods, such as yogurt, miso, and sauerkraut. It has been shown to have extremely positive effects in the digestive tract, where the balance of good and bad bacteria is the foundation of the body's ability to fight bacterial infection, viruses, and fungal overgrowths. Kefir has also been shown to destroy harmful invading bacteria, and is believed to slow the growth of certain tumors. One of the probiotic bacteria alive in kefir, *Lactobacillus casei*, is strong enough to fight off pneumonia.

- Kefir's smaller curds make it easier to digest than yogurt, which helps it in its task of removing toxins via the digestive tract.
- Has all the protein and calcium benefits of milk but is easier to tolerate for people with mild lactose intolerance.
- Traditionally used to boost energy, help relieve skin disorders, and promote longevity.

Practical tips:
You can find kefir at good health-food stores, or make it yourself from cultures available on the Internet. Kefir can also be made with coconut water or even just water (although the nutritional values listed on this page include the nutrients of milk). Use kefir as you would yogurt. It makes a great base for smoothies because the sour taste offsets fruit perfectly.

BLUEBERRY SMOOTHIE

SERVES 2

½ cup kefir
½ cup water
1½ cups blueberries

METHOD

1 Put the kefir, water, and blueberries into a food processor or blender and process until smooth.

2 Pour into glasses and serve immediately.

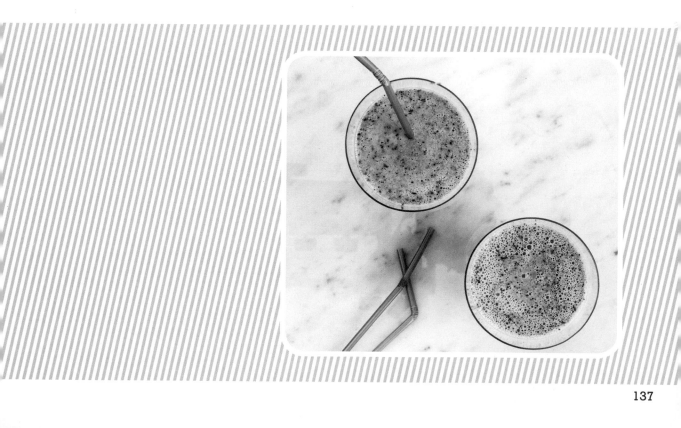

KEFIR BREAD

MAKES 1 LARGE LOAF

2¼ teaspoons fast-action yeast

¾ cup lukewarm water

3¾ cups white bread flour, plus extra for dusting

1½ teaspoons fine sea salt

1 teaspoon superfine sugar

⅔ cup kefir milk, plus extra for glazing

olive oil, for greasing

a little polenta or semolina for sprinkling

METHOD

1   Sprinkle the yeast over the warm water, stir and set aside for 10 minutes. In a large bowl sift together the flour, salt, and sugar. Create a well in the centre and pour in the yeast mixture, and kefir milk. Mix to a wet dough, then tip onto a flour-dusted work surface and knead for 10 minutes, until smooth and elastic. Shape into a ball and place in a large lightly oiled bowl. Cover with plastic wrap and leave in a warm place for 30 minutes.

2   Knead the dough briefly for about a minute then shape back into a ball and place back in the bowl, re-cover and set aside for an additional 30 minutes, or until doubled in size.

3   Dust a baking sheet with polenta. Shape the dough into an oval and place on the baking sheet. Cover loosely with lightly oiled plastic wrap and set aside for 30 minutes. Preheat a second baking sheet in the oven to 425°F.

4   Brush the loaf all over in kefir and slash a line down the middle with a serrated knife. Place on top of the preheated baking sheet and bake for 40 minutes, or until golden with a firm crust. Cool on a wire rack before serving.

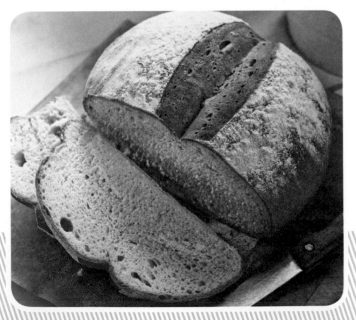

KEFIR PASTRY PARCELS

MAKES 15

2 cups all-purpose flour, plus extra for dusting

pinch of salt

½ cup confectioners' sugar

1¼ sticks unsalted cold butter, chopped

3 tablespoons kefir milk

1 ounce ground almonds

1 large egg, beaten, for brushing

granulated sugar, for sprinkling

FILLING

7 ounces ripe blackberries

2 tablespoons superfine sugar

2 teaspoons lemon juice

2 tablespoons raspberry preserves

METHOD

1 In a food processor, mix the flour, salt, and sugar. Add the butter and pulse until the mixture resembles fine bread crumbs. Add the kefir milk and pulse again so that the pastry dough comes together in large lumps. Knead briefly, then wrap in plastic wrap and chill in the refrigerator for at least 30 minutes.

2 Meanwhile, to make the filling, put the blackberries into a bowl with the sugar and lemon juice, and crush lightly. Stir through the preserves.

3 Preheat a baking sheet in the oven to 400°F. Roll the pastry dough out on a lightly floured surface, to ¼-inch thick, and stamp out 15 rounds using a 3½-inch round cookie cutter, re-rolling trimmings if needed. Sprinkle each pastry round with 1 teaspoon of ground almonds, then place a spoonful of the blackberry filling into the middle of each. Brush the sides of the pastry with egg and fold the pastry over to enclose. Pinch the edges to seal.

4 Place the pastry parcels on a baking sheet lined with baking parchment. Brush the tops all over with beaten egg and sprinkle with granulated sugar. Bake in the preheated oven for 20–25 minutes, until golden. Serve warm.

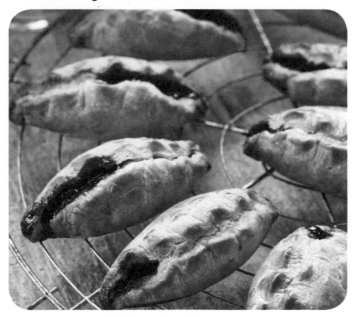

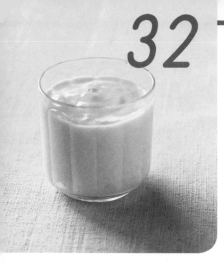

32

GREEK YOGURT

Greek yogurt with live cultures contains bacterial cultures that boost the immune system and keep the digestive system healthy and robust.

MAJOR NUTRIENTS PER ½ CUP GREEK YOGURT (WITH LIVE CULTURES)

Calories	61
Total fat	3.25g
Protein	3.47g
Carbohydrate	4.66g
Vitamin A	99 IU
Vitamin B2	0.14mg
Vitamin B5	0.39mg
Vitamin B12	0.37mcg
Choline	15.2mg
Calcium	121mg
Potassium	155mg

Greek yogurt contains less sugar and more protein than other yogurts because it is strained to remove the carbohydrate-rich whey. Its thick texture leaves you fuller than more watery versions and the lower level of lactose (milk sugar) it contains makes it easier to digest. Eating yogurt with live cultures regularly has been shown to enhance immune responses and improve resistance to disease.

• All yogurt helps reduce bad cholesterol, but only yogurt with live cultures raises good cholesterol levels, making sure the arteries stay healthy.
• An important vitamin B12 source for vegetarians, which could help to prevent skin conditions, as well as Alzheimer's disease, heart disease, and diabetes.

Practical tips:
Always choose yogurt with live cultures for the beneficial bacterial cultures. If possible, buy from local farms via health-food stores or farmer's markets—these products will have their own natural bacteria instead of bacteria that has been added in the production process. Avoid fruit-flavored yogurt, because it often contains added sugar; instead, sweeten the yogurt with fresh fruit or cinnamon. The creamy, fresh taste of Greek yogurt makes it a good alternative to milk, cream, sour cream, and crème fraîche in main meals and side dishes, as well as some desserts.

TZATZIKI

SERVES 4

1 small cucumber

1¼ cups Greek yogurt with live cultures

1 large garlic clove, crushed

1 tablespoon chopped fresh mint or dill

salt and pepper, to taste

METHOD

1 Peel and grate the cucumber. Put in a strainer and squeeze out as much of the water as possible. Put the cucumber into a bowl.

2 Add the yogurt, garlic, and chopped mint (reserve a little as a garnish, if desired) to the cucumber and season with pepper. Mix well together and chill in the refrigerator for about 2 hours before serving.

3 Stir the dip and transfer to a serving bowl. Sprinkle with salt and serve garnished with chopped mint, if desired.

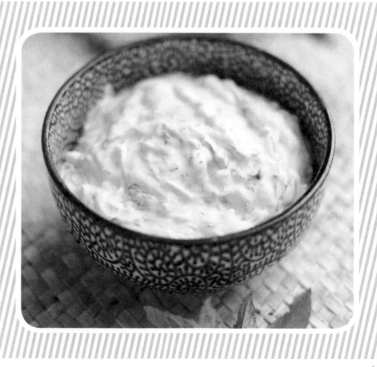

RED CABBAGE & BEET SLAW

SERVES 4

3¾ cups finely shredded red cabbage

1 cup julienned cooked beets

1 apple, cored and thinly sliced

1 tablespoon lemon juice

1 tablespoon sunflower seeds

1 tablespoon pumpkin seeds

DRESSING

3 tablespoons mayonnaise

4 tablespoons Greek yogurt

1 tablespoon red wine vinegar

salt and pepper, to taste

METHOD

1   Put the cabbage, beets, and apple slices into a large bowl. Add the lemon juice and mix well.

2   To make the dressing, mix all of the dressing ingredients together in a separate bowl. Pour the dressing over the salad and stir well. Season with salt and pepper, cover, and chill in the refrigerator for at least 1 hour.

3   Stir the salad thoroughly and adjust the seasoning to taste. Sprinkle with the sunflower and pumpkin seeds just before serving.

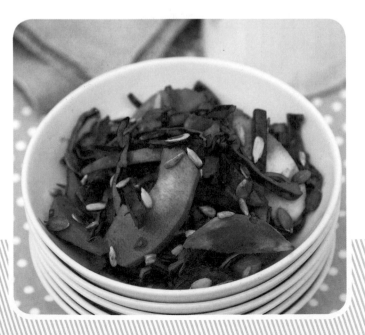

HERBED FETA DIP

SERVES 4-6

1 cup feta cheese, crumbled

¼ cup Greek yogurt

2 tablespoons extra virgin olive oil

rind and juice of 1 small lemon

small bunch of fresh mint, chopped

small bunch of fresh flat-leaf parsley, chopped

½ red chile, seeded and chopped

pepper, to taste

METHOD

1 Put the cheese, yogurt, and oil in a food processor and process for 30 seconds, until combined.

2 Scrape the mixture into a bowl and then add the lemon rind and juice, mint, parsley, and chile. Season with pepper to taste and mix well.

3 Place in the refrigerator to chill for 30 minutes before serving.

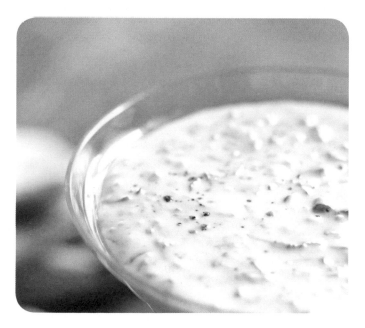

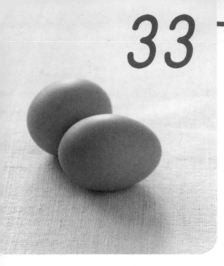

33

EGGS

Eggs are an excellent source of protein, and they also contain all of the amino acids necessary for the body to repair and regenerate cells.

Eggs are ideally packaged to support new life, and so contain all the nutrients we need for growth: iron, zinc, vitamin A, vitamin D, the B vitamins, and omega-3 fats. Many people avoid them because of their high cholesterol content, but the body can regulate this if the diet is generally low in sugar and saturated fat. Many studies show that egg consumption helps prevent chronic age-related conditions, such as coronary heart disease, loss of muscle mass, eye degeneration, hearing loss, and memory loss.

- Contain vitamin B12 to help combat fatigue, depression, and lethargy.
- Vitamin A and lutein ensure eye protection and continuing good sight.
- One of the few dietary sources of both vitamins K and D, which work together to keep bones strong.
- Contain sulfur and lecithin, substances that help the liver with digestion and detoxification.

Practical tips:
Eggs are a truly useful staple food—they can be cooked in many different ways, including poaching, scrambling, and boiling. Omelets or frittatas, loaded with healthy vegetables, can also be eaten cold as a snack. Buy organic eggs from pasture-raised chickens because their feed gives these eggs higher nutritional value, indicated by their deeper-yellow yolk and richer taste.

MAJOR NUTRIENTS PER MEDIUM EGG

Calories	65
Total fat	4.37g
Omega-3 oils	32.6mg
Omega-6 oils	505mg
Omega-9 oils	1,582mg
Protein	5.53g
Carbohydrate	0.34g
Vitamin A	214 IU
Vitamin D	22 IU
Vitamin B2	0.21mg
Vitamin B5	0.63mg
Vitamin B12	0.57mcg
Vitamin K	0.1mcg
Choline	110.5mg
Iron	0.81mg
Selenium	13.9mcg
Zinc	0.49mg
Lutein/Zeaxanthin	146mcg

MIXED HERB OMELET

SERVES 1

2 extra-large eggs
2 tablespoons milk
3 tablespoons butter
leaves from 1 fresh parsley
sprig, chopped
2 fresh chives, snipped
salt and pepper, to taste
fresh salad greens, to serve

METHOD

1 Break the eggs into a bowl. Add the milk and season with salt and pepper, then quickly beat until just blended.

2 Heat a skillet over medium–high heat until hot. Add 2 tablespoons of the butter and use a spatula to rub it over the bottom and around the side of the skillet as it melts.

3 As soon as the butter stops sizzling, pour in the eggs. Use the spatula to stir the eggs around the skillet in a circular motion. Do not scrape the bottom of the skillet.

4 As the omelet begins to set, use the spatula to push the cooked egg toward the center of the skillet. Continue doing this for 3 minutes, or until the omelet looks set on the bottom but is still slightly runny on top.

5 Put the chopped herbs in the center of the omelet. Use the spatula to fold the omelet in half, over the herbs. Slide onto a plate, then rub the remaining butter over the top. Serve immediately, accompanied by fresh salad greens.

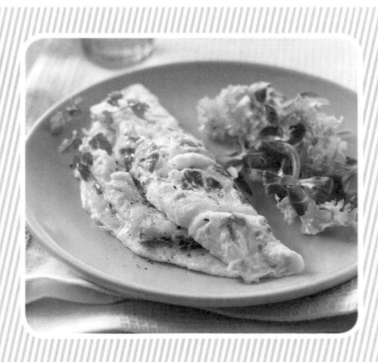

\KED EGGS WITH \TOMATO & CORN SAUCE

SERVES 4

2 tablespoons butter

2 tablespoons olive oil

1 onion, finely chopped

2 garlic cloves, finely chopped

1 celery stalk, finely chopped

8 ounces lean bacon, diced

1 red bell pepper, seeded and diced

4 plum tomatoes, peeled, cored, and chopped

2 tablespoons tomato paste

brown sugar, to taste

1 tablespoon chopped fresh parsley

pinch of cayenne pepper

1 (8½-ounce) can corn kernels, drained

4 extra-large eggs

salt and pepper, to taste

METHOD

1   Melt the butter with the oil in a saucepan. Add the onion, garlic, and celery and cook over low heat, stirring occasionally, for 5 minutes, until softened. Add the bacon and red bell pepper and cook, stirring occasionally, for an additional 10 minutes.

2   Stir in the tomatoes, tomato paste, sugar, parsley, cayenne, and ½ cup of water and season with salt and pepper. Increase the heat to medium and bring to a boil, then reduce the heat and simmer, stirring occasionally, for 15 minutes, until thickened. Meanwhile, preheat the oven to 350°F.

3   Stir the corn kernels into the sauce and transfer the mixture to an ovenproof dish. Make four small hollows with the back of a spoon and break an egg into each. Bake in the preheated oven for 25–30 minutes, until the eggs have set. Serve.

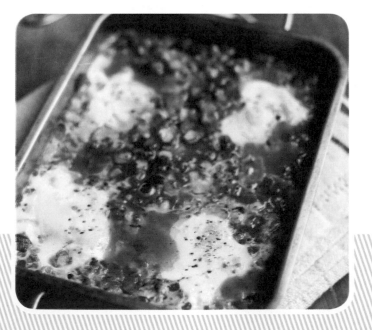

POACHED EGGS FLORENTINE

SERVES 4

1 tablespoon olive oil
1 (6-ounce) package fresh spinach
4 thick slices ciabatta bread
2 tablespoons butter
4 extra-large eggs
1 cup shredded cheddar cheese
salt and pepper, to taste
freshly grated nutmeg, to serve

METHOD

1 Preheat the broiler to high. Heat the oil in a large saucepan, add the spinach, and sauté for 2–3 minutes, until the leaves are wilted. Drain in a colander, squeezing out as much water with the back of a wooden spoon. Season with salt and pepper, and keep warm.

2 Toast the bread on both sides until golden. Spread one side of each slice with butter and place buttered-side up on a baking sheet.

3 Bring a small saucepan of lightly salted water to a boil, crack the eggs into the water, and poach for about 3 minutes, until the whites are set but the yolks still runny. Remove from the pan with a slotted spoon.

4 Arrange the spinach on the toast and top each slice with a poached egg. Sprinkle with the shredded cheese. Cook under the preheated broiler for 1–2 minutes, until the cheese has melted. Sprinkle with nutmeg and serve.

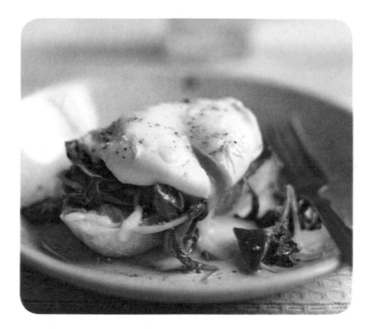

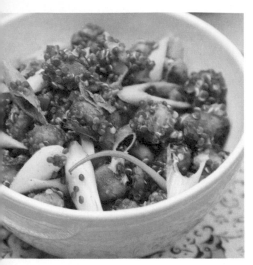

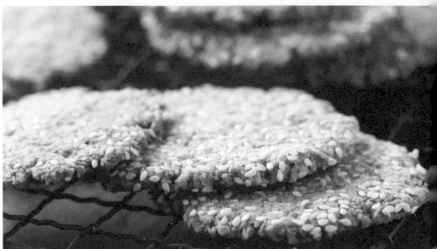

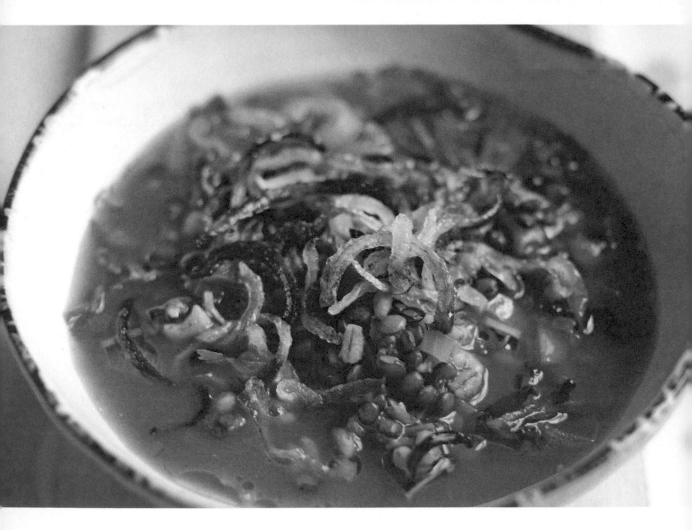

GRAINS & PULSES

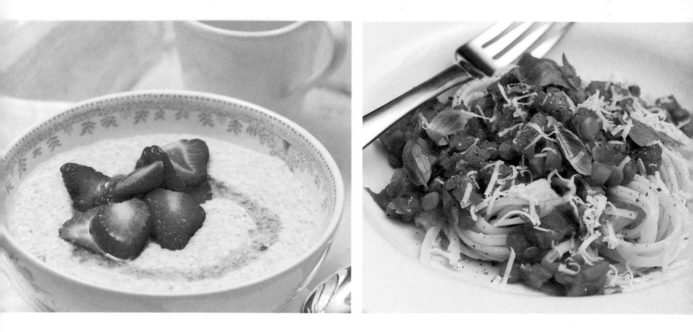

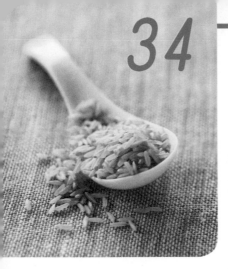

34

BROWN RICE

The high fiber content of brown rice can help lower blood cholesterol levels and keep blood-sugar levels even, making it a healthier choice than white rice.

While white rice contains few nutrients other than starch, brown rice has several nutritional benefits. Regular consumption of brown rice and other whole grains has been shown to help prevent heart disease, diabetes, and some cancers. It is a good source of fiber, which can help reduce cholesterol levels and keep blood-sugar levels even. Brown rice also contains some protein, and is a good source of several of the B vitamins and of minerals, particularly selenium and magnesium.

- A reasonably low glycemic index (GI) food that can help control blood-sugar levels and may be helpful for diabetics.
- Useful B vitamin content to help convert food into energy and keep the nervous system healthy.
- High selenium content may help protect against cancers, and high magnesium content is important for a healthy heart.

Practical tips:
Store rice in a cool, dark cupboard and use within a few months of purchase. Brown rice tends not to keep as well as white rice because it contains small amounts of fat, which can spoil over time. It's also worth noting that the longer you store raw rice, the longer it may take to cook. Leftover cooked rice can be kept for a day or two in a refrigerator if you cool it quickly, but it must be reheated until piping hot before serving to kill bacteria that can cause food poisoning.

MAJOR NUTRIENTS PER ⅓ CUP/2½ OUNCES BROWN RICE, UNCOOKED

Calories	222
Total fat	1.8g
Protein	5g
Carbohydrate	46g
Fiber	3.6g
Niacin	3mg
Vitamin B1	0.2mg
Vitamin B6	0.3mg
Selenium	19.6mcg
Magnesium	86mg
Iron	0.8mg
Zinc	1.3g
Calcium	20mg

DID YOU KNOW?

Ninety percent of all rice is still grown and consumed in Asia, where it has been eaten for over 6,000 years.

MULLIGATAWNY SOUP

SERVES 4–6

½ cup butter

2 onions, chopped

1 small turnip, cut into small dice

2 carrots, finely sliced

1 apple, peeled, cored, and chopped

2 tablespoons mild curry powder

5 cups chicken stock

juice of ½ lemon

6 ounces cold cooked chicken, chopped

2 tablespoons chopped fresh cilantro, plus extra to garnish

salt and pepper, to taste

½ cup cooked rice, to serve

METHOD

1 Melt the butter in a large saucepan over medium heat. Add the onions and sauté gently, until soft but not brown.

2 Add the turnip, carrots, and apple and continue to cook for an additional 3–4 minutes.

3 Stir in the curry powder until the vegetables are well coated, then pour in the stock. Bring to a boil, cover, and simmer for about 45 minutes. Season to taste with salt and pepper and add the lemon juice.

4 Transfer the soup to a food processor or blender. Process until smooth and return to the rinsed-out saucepan. Add the chicken and cilantro to the pan and reheat gently.

5 Remove the soup from the heat. Divide the rice among warmed bowls and ladle the soup over the top. Garnish with cilantro and serve immediately.

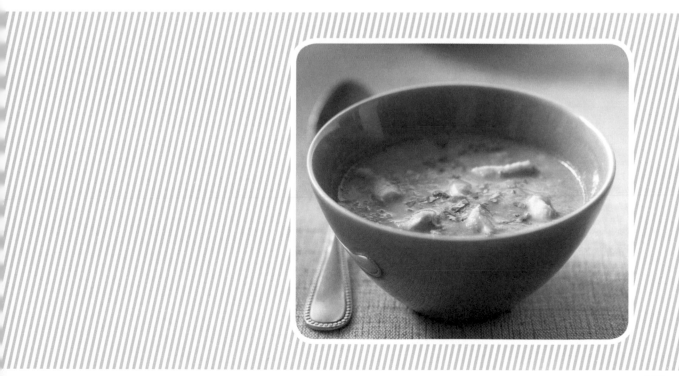

BROWN RICE LUNCHBOWL

SERVES 4

1¼ cups brown long-grain rice

1 bay leaf

2½ cups gluten-free vegetable stock or water

8 ounces asparagus, cut into 1¼-inch pieces

juice of 1 lime

2 tablespoons extra virgin olive oil

½ cup coarsely chopped Brazil nuts

salt and pepper, to taste

METHOD

1 Put the rice and bay leaf in a large saucepan with the stock over high heat and bring to a boil. Stir lightly, then reduce the heat. Cover and simmer, stirring occasionally, for about 35 minutes, or according to the package directions, until all the liquid is absorbed and the rice is just tender. Remove and discard the bay leaf.

2 Meanwhile, bring a saucepan of water to a boil over high heat. Add the asparagus and boil for 3–5 minutes, or until just tender. Alternatively, steam the asparagus for 5–6 minutes over boiling water to preserve more nutrients. Drain well.

3 Combine the rice and asparagus in a large bowl and pour the lime juice and olive oil over the top. Mix well to combine thoroughly.

4 Stir in the Brazil nuts and season with salt and pepper. Serve warm or cold.

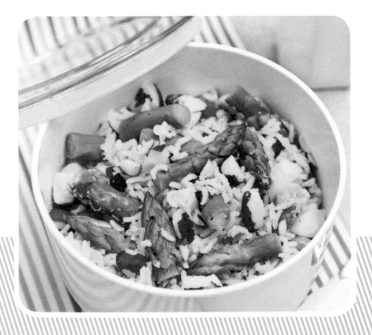

SPICY CHICKPEA & BROWN RICE SALAD

SERVES 4

½ tablespoon olive oil

1 teaspoon cumin seeds, gently crushed

½ teaspoon coriander seeds, gently crushed

1 red onion, sliced

¾ teaspoon garam masala (available in Asian grocery stores, or make your own by mixing equal parts ground cumin, black pepper, cloves, and nutmeg)

1½ cups brown rice

⅓ cup raisins

3½ cups simmering vegetable stock

1 (15-ounce) can chickpeas, drained and rinsed

⅓ cup chopped fresh cilantro, plus extra sprigs to garnish

2 tablespoons slivered almonds

1⅓ cups drained and crumbled feta cheese, to serve

METHOD

1   Heat the olive oil in a saucepan and add the cumin and coriander seeds. Cook for a minute before adding the onion. Sauté the onion for 2–3 minutes, then stir in the garam masala. Stir in the rice and raisins, making sure they are coated with the spices.

2   Pour in the stock and bring to a boil. Reduce the heat, then cover and simmer for 25 minutes, until all the stock is absorbed and the rice is cooked.

3   Stir in the drained chickpeas, cilantro, and slivered almonds. Remove from the heat, transfer to serving bowls, and serve, warm, or cold, topped with crumbled feta cheese and garnished with fresh cilantro.

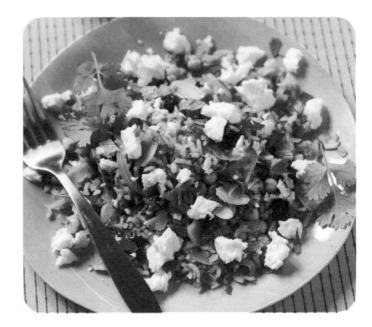

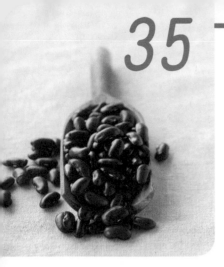

35

KIDNEY BEANS

Iron-rich kidney beans are an excellent source of good-quality protein, zinc, and fiber, and they contain compounds that help prevent blood clots.

Kidney beans are invaluable for vegetarians because they are high in good-quality protein and minerals. A ⅓ cup/2¼-ounce portion of kidney beans contains at least one-quarter of our day's iron needs to help prevent anemia and increase energy levels, while their good zinc content helps boost the immune system and maintain fertility. The high degree of insoluble fiber in kidney beans helps prevent colon cancer, while for diabetics and people with insulin resistance, the total fiber content helps to regulate blood-sugar levels.

- Excellent source of protein, iron, and calcium for vegetarians.
- Very high fiber content helps regulate release of insulin and helps to prevent hunger—a good choice for dieters.
- Protects against colon cancer.
- Extremely high in potassium, which can minimize fluid retention and may help control high blood pressure.

Practical tips:
There is little nutritional difference between cooked dried kidney beans and canned kidney beans, so, if you don't have much time, use canned beans. Raw kidney beans contain a toxin that can cause an upset stomach, vomiting, and diarrhea if not cooked correctly. When using dried beans, they must be soaked overnight, or for at least 12 hours, and then rinsed in fresh cold water before being rapidly boiled for at least 10 minutes before cooking to remove the toxins.

MAJOR NUTRIENTS PER
⅓ CUP/2¼ OUNCES DRIED
RED KIDNEY BEANS

Calories	200
Total fat	0.8g
Protein	13.7g
Carbohydrate	36g
Fiber	10g
Folate	205mcg
Vitamin B1	0.25mg
Niacin	0.9mg
Magnesium	66mg
Potassium	640mg
Zinc	1.6g
Calcium	55mg
Iron	3.5mg

MIXED BEAN CHILI

SERVES 5

1 cup dried mixed beans, such as red kidney, pinto, cannellini, and chickpeas

1 red onion, diced

1 garlic clove, crushed

1 tablespoon hot chili powder

1 (14½-ounce) can diced tomatoes

1 tablespoon tomato paste

¼ cup low-fat plain yogurt, to garnish

soft flour tortilla wraps, to serve

METHOD

1. Soak the beans overnight in a large bowl of cold water. Drain, rinse, and put the beans into a large saucepan. Cover with cold water, then bring to a boil and boil rapidly for 10 minutes. Reduce the heat, cover, and simmer for an additional 45 minutes, or until tender. Drain.

2. Put the cooked beans, onion, garlic, chili powder, tomatoes, and tomato paste into a saucepan and bring to a boil. Reduce the heat, cover, and simmer for 20–25 minutes, or until the onion is tender.

3. Ladle the chili into bowls and top each bowl with some of the yogurt. Serve immediately with soft flour tortilla wraps.

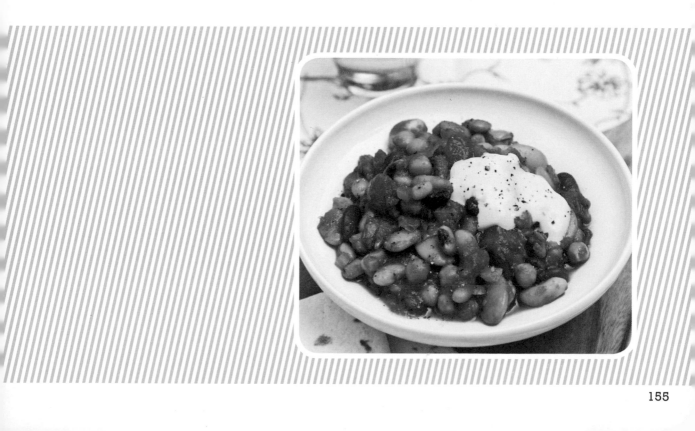

RED BEANS & RICE

MAKES 6

1 pound dried red kidney beans, soaked in water overnight

1 pound smoked ham hocks

2 cups chopped onion

2 cups chopped celery

2 cups chopped green bell pepper

¼ cup chopped fresh parsley

1 (8-ounce) can tomato sauce

3 bay leaves

1 teaspoon dried thyme

1 teaspoon garlic powder

1 teaspoon dried oregano leaves

1 teaspoon cayenne pepper

½-1 teaspoon hot sauce

1 pound smoked sausage

salt and pepper, to taste

cooked rice, to serve

METHOD

1 Drain and rinse the beans, place in a large dutch oven and cover with fresh cold water. Add all of the remaining ingredients, except the sausage; bring to a boil over high heat. Season to taste with salt and pepper, then cover, reduce the heat, and simmer for 1 hour and 45 minutes.

2 Remove the ham hocks, and set aside. Cut the sausage into ½-inch pieces and add to the dutch oven. Cook, uncovered, over low heat for 40 minutes, stirring occasionally. Remove and discard the bay leaves.

3 Remove any meat from the ham hocks and add to the dutch oven. Stir well and cook, uncovered, until heated through. Serve over cooked rice.

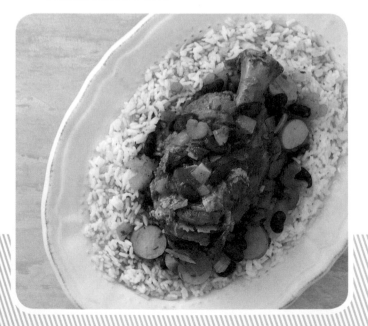

VEGETARIAN CHILE BURGERS

SERVES 4–6

½ cup bulgur wheat

1 cup drained, rinsed canned red kidney beans

1 cup drained, rinsed canned cannellini beans

1–2 fresh red jalapeño chiles, seeded and coarsely chopped

2–3 garlic cloves

6 scallions, coarsely chopped

1 yellow bell pepper, seeded, peeled and chopped

1 tablespoon chopped fresh cilantro

1 cup shredded cheddar cheese or Monterey Jack cheese

2 tablespoons whole-wheat flour

1–2 tablespoons sunflower oil

1 large tomato, sliced

salt and pepper

whole-wheat buns, to serve

METHOD

1 Place the bulgur wheat in a strainer and rinse under cold running water. Cook the bulgur wheat in a saucepan of lightly salted water according to the package directions, until tender. Drain and reserve.

2 Place the beans in a food processor with the chiles, garlic, scallions, yellow bell pepper, cilantro, and half the cheese. Using the pulse button, chop finely. Add to the cooked bulgur wheat and season with salt and pepper. Mix well, then shape into four to six equal burgers. Cover and let chill for 1 hour. Coat the burgers in the flour.

3 Preheat the broiler to medium. Heat a heavy skillet and add the oil. When hot, add the burgers and cook over medium heat for 5–6 minutes on each side, or until piping hot.

4 Place one to two slices of tomato on top of each burger and sprinkle with the remaining cheese. Cook under the hot broiler for 2–3 minutes, or until the cheese begins to melt. Serve in whole wheat buns.

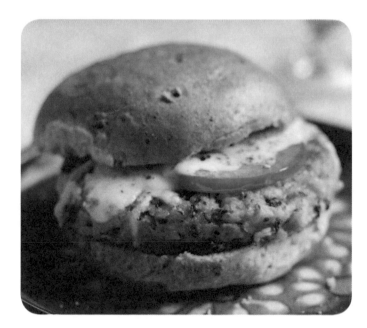

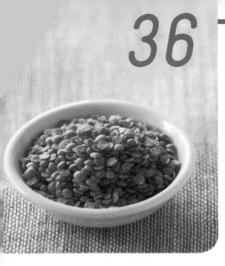

36

LENTILS

Small, lens-shaped dried lentils are one of the beans richest in cancer-blocking fibers called isoflavones and lignan, and they are low in fat and saturates.

Lentils come in a variety of colors and include green, brown, and red. Green and brown lentils tend to contain the highest levels of nutrients and fiber. Lentils are a rich source of fiber, both insoluble and soluble, which helps protect us against cancer and cardiovascular disease. They also contain plant chemicals called isoflavones, which may offer protection from cancer and coronary heart disease, and lignan, which has a mild estrogen-like effect that may lower the risk of cancer, minimize premenstrual syndrome, and protect against osteoporosis. Lentils are also rich in the B vitamins, folate, and all major minerals, particularly iron and zinc.

- Rich in fiber for protection from cardiovascular disease and cancers.
- High iron content for healthy blood and energy levels.
- Contain plant chemicals to help premenstrual syndrome and bone health.
- High zinc content to boost the immune system.

Practical tips:
Lentils are one of the few dried beans that don't need soaking before cooking. They are also relatively quick to cook, and will take approximately 30 minutes in simmering water. Cooking dried lentils in stock makes a simple, healthy base for a soup, which can be added to as desired. Canned lentils have almost as many nutrients as dried ones so are a convenient alternative.

MAJOR NUTRIENTS PER 1/3 CUP/2¼ OUNCES DRIED RED LENTILS

Calories	212
Total fat	0.6g
Protein	15.5g
Carbohydrate	36g
Fiber	18g
Folate	287mcg
Vitamin B1	0.5mg
Niacin	1.6mg
Vitamin B6	0.3mg
Magnesium	73mg
Potassium	573mg
Zinc	2.9g
Calcium	34mg
Iron	4.5mg

DID YOU KNOW?

Lentils are thought to be one of the earliest foods to have been cultivated, with 8,000-year old-seeds found at sites in the Middle East.

FIVE-SPICE LENTIL STEW

SERVES 4

⅔ cup dried red split lentils

⅔ cup dried peeled, split mung beans

3¾ cups hot water

1 teaspoon ground turmeric

1 teaspoon salt, or to taste

1 tablespoon lemon juice

2 tablespoons olive oil

¼ teaspoon black mustard seeds

¼ teaspoon cumin seeds

¼ teaspoon nigella seeds

¼ teaspoon fennel seeds

4–5 fenugreek seeds

2–3 crushed red peppers

1 small tomato, seeded and cut into strips and fresh cilantro sprigs, to garnish

METHOD

1 Rinse the lentils and mung beans under cold running water, then place in a saucepan with the hot water and bring to a boil. Reduce the heat and simmer for 5–6 minutes. Add the turmeric, reduce the heat to low, cover, and cook for an additional 20 minutes. Add the salt, lemon juice, and a little more water if the mixture is too thick.

2 Heat the oil in a small saucepan over medium heat. When hot, but not smoking, add the mustard seeds. As soon as they begin to pop, reduce the heat to low and add the cumin seeds, nigella seeds, fennel seeds, fenugreek seeds, and crushed red pepper. Let the spices sizzle until the seeds begin to pop and the crushed pepper has blackened.

3 Transfer to a serving dish and pour the contents of the saucepan over the lentils. Garnish with the tomato strips and cilantro sprigs. Serve immediately.

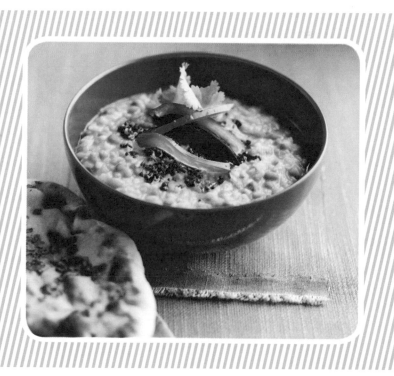

SPICED LENTIL BURGER

MAKES 6

½ cup green lentils

1 carrot, peeled and diced

2 tablespoons vegetable oil, plus extra for frying

1 tablespoon brown mustard seeds

1 teaspoon ground coriander

1 teaspoon ground cumin

½ onion, finely chopped

1 teaspoon minced garlic

1 fresh serrano chile, finely chopped

⅓ cup frozen peas, thawed

1 potato, cooked and mashed

1¼ cups fresh bread crumbs

6 whole-wheat hamburger buns, halved

store-bought mango chutney

lettuce leaves

salt and pepper, to taste

METHOD

1 Bring a large saucepan of lightly salted water to a boil. Add the lentils, bring back to a boil, then reduce the heat and simmer for 15 minutes. Add the carrot and cook for about 10 minutes, until the lentils are soft. Drain.

2 Heat the oil in a medium sauté pan. Add the mustard seeds, coriander, and cumin and swirl to coat in the oil. Add the onion, garlic, and chile and cook for 5–8 minutes, stirring frequently, until the onion is soft. Stir in the lentils and carrot and simmer for about 5 minutes to evaporate any liquid. Add the peas and potato and season with salt and pepper, then combine thoroughly.

3 Place the bread crumbs in a shallow bowl. Scoop out the lentil mixture in six equal portions and shape each portion into a patty. Press each patty in the bread crumbs to cover both sides.

4 Place a ridged grill pan or large skillet over medium heat and add enough oil to coat the bottom. Add the patties and cook for about 5 minutes on each side until brown.

5 Place the burgers in the buns, top with the chutney and lettuce leaves, and serve immediately.

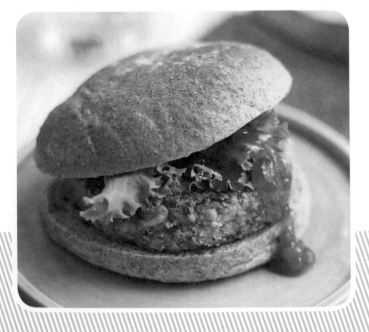

SPAGHETTI WITH LENTIL & TOMATO SAUCE

SERVES 4

1 cup dried green lentils

2 tablespoons olive oil

1 large onion, chopped

2 garlic cloves, crushed

2 carrots, chopped

2 celery stalks, chopped

1 (28-ounce) can diced tomatoes

⅔ cup vegetable stock

1 red bell pepper, seeded and chopped

2 tablespoons tomato paste

2 teaspoons finely chopped fresh rosemary

1 teaspoon dried oregano

10 ounces dried spaghetti or linguine

handful of basil leaves, torn

salt and pepper

freshly grated vegetarian Parmesan-style cheese, to serve

METHOD

1 Put the lentils in a saucepan and cover with cold water. Bring to a boil and simmer for about 30 minutes, or according to the package directions, until just tender. Drain well.

2 Meanwhile, heat the oil in a large saucepan. Add the onion, garlic, carrots, and celery. Cover and cook over low heat for 5 minutes. Stir in the tomatoes, stock, red bell pepper, tomato paste, rosemary, and oregano. Cover and simmer for 20 minutes, until the sauce is thickened and the vegetables are tender. Add the lentils and cook, stirring, for an additional 5 minutes. Season with salt and pepper.

3 While the sauce is cooking, bring a large saucepan of lightly salted water to a boil. Add the spaghetti, bring back to a boil, and cook according to the package directions, until tender but still firm to the bite. Drain well, then divide the spaghetti among four warm bowls. Spoon the sauce over the pasta and sprinkle with the basil leaves. Serve immediately with the grated cheese on the side.

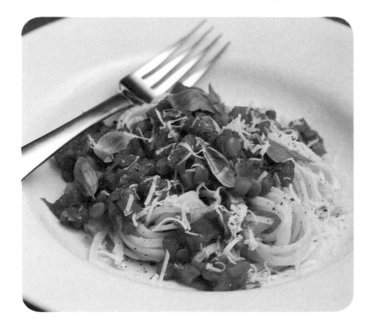

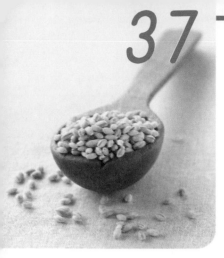

37

POT BARLEY

This extremely nutritious starchy grain contains soluble fiber, which helps to lower bad blood cholesterol and protects from hormonal cancers and heart disease.

***MAJOR NUTRIENTS PER
⅓ CUP/2¼ OUNCES
POT BARLEY, UNCOOKED***

Calories	212
Total fat	1.4g
Protein	7.5g
Carbohydrate	44g
Fiber	10.4g
Vitamin B1	0.4mg
Niacin	2.8mg
Selenium	22.5mcg
Magnesium	80mg
Potassium	271mg
Zinc	1.7g
Calcium	20mg
Iron	2.2mg
Lutein/Zeaxanthin	96mcg

Pot barley is a grain with a rich, slightly nutty flavor and a chewy texture. Most barley that is sold is pearl barley, which has had some of the nutrients and fiber removed, by processing, whereas pot barley has been polished so only the hull has been removed and is therefore a good source of nutrients. These include a fiber-like compound called lignan, which may protect against breast and other hormone-dependent cancers, as well as heart disease. Unusually for a grain, barley contains lutein and zeaxanthin, both of which help to protect eyesight and eye health.

• Whole grain that protects against cancers and heart disease.
• A good source of minerals and the B vitamins.
• High in fiber to keep the colon healthy and soluble fiber to lower blood cholesterol.
• Helps to keep eyes healthy.

Practical tips:
Pot barley needs up to two hours of simmering in water, but presoaking it for several hours will shorten the cooking time. The fats in barley can make it spoil after a short time, especially if kept in warm, light conditions, so store barley in a cool, dry, dark place in an airtight container and use within two to three months. Barley water, made by steeping the grains in water, has long been considered a health drink for its diuretic and kidney-supporting effect.

HEARTY BARLEY VEGETABLE SOUP

SERVES 4–6

2 tablespoons sunflower oil
1 onion, finely chopped
1 celery stalk, finely chopped
1 garlic clove, crushed
6½ cups vegetable stock
½ cup pot barley, rinsed
1 bouquet garni, made with 1 bay leaf, fresh thyme sprigs, and fresh parsley sprigs tied together
2 carrots, peeled and diced
1 (14½-ounce) can diced tomatoes
½ head cabbage, cored and shredded
salt and pepper, to taste
2 tablespoons chopped fresh parsley, to garnish

METHOD

1   Heat the oil in a large saucepan. Add the onion, celery, and garlic and cook over medium heat for 5–7 minutes, or until softened.

2   Pour in the stock and bring to a boil, skimming off any foam that rises to the surface with a slotted spoon. Add the barley and bouquet garni, reduce the heat to low, cover, and simmer for 30 minutes–1 hour, or until the grains are just beginning to soften.

3   Add the carrots, and tomatoes with their can juices to the pan. Bring the liquid back to a boil, then reduce the heat to low, cover, and simmer for an additional 30 minutes, or until the barley and carrots are tender.

4   Just before serving, remove the bouquet garni, stir in the cabbage, and season with salt and pepper. Cook until the cabbage wilts, then ladle into warm soup bowls, garnish with parsley, and serve immediately.

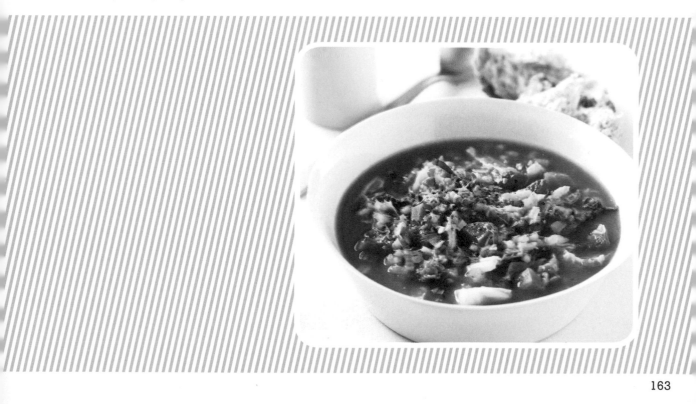

CHICKEN & BARLEY STEW

SERVES 4

2 tablespoons vegetable oil

8 small skinless chicken thighs

2½ cups chicken stock

½ cup pearl barley, rinsed and drained

7 ounces small new potatoes, scrubbed and halved lengthways

2 large carrots, sliced

1 leek, sliced

2 shallots, sliced

1 tablespoon tomato paste

1 bay leaf

1 zucchini, sliced

2 tablespoons chopped fresh flat-leaf parsley

2 tablespoons plain flour

4 tablespoons water

salt and pepper, to taste

METHOD

1 Heat the oil in a large saucepan over medium heat. Add the chicken and cook for 3 minutes, then turn over and cook on the other side for a further 2 minutes. Add the stock, pearl barley, potatoes, carrots, leek, shallots, tomato paste, and bay leaf. Bring to a boil, reduce the heat and simmer for 30 minutes.

2 Add the zucchini and chopped parsley, cover the pan and cook for a further 20 minutes, or until the chicken is tender and the juices run clear when a skewer is inserted into the thickest part of the meat. Remove and discard the bay leaf.

3 In a bowl, mix the flour with the water and stir to a smooth paste. Add it to the stew and cook, stirring, over a low heat for an additional 5 minutes. Season to taste with salt and pepper.

4 Remove from the heat, ladle into individual serving bowls and garnish with parsley sprigs. Serve immediately.

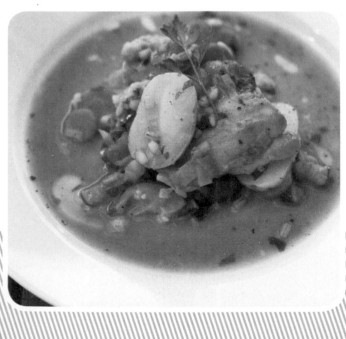

BARLEY, LENTIL & ONION SOUP

SERVES 6

2 tablespoons pearl barley

⅔ cup water

7 cups vegetable stock

3 onions, thinly sliced into rings

¾ cup dried green lentils

½ teaspoon ground ginger

1 teaspoon ground cumin

3 tablespoons lemon juice

2 tablespoons chopped fresh cilantro

salt and pepper, to taste

TO GARNISH

2 onions, halved and thinly sliced

⅓ cup vegetable oil

2 garlic cloves, finely chopped

METHOD

1 Put the barley into a large saucepan, pour in the water, and bring to a boil. Reduce the heat, cover, and simmer gently, stirring frequently, for about 30 minutes, until all the liquid has been absorbed.

2 Add the stock, onions, lentils, ginger, and cumin and bring to a boil over medium heat. Reduce the heat, cover, and simmer, stirring occasionally, for 1½ hours, adding a little more stock, if necessary.

3 Meanwhile, make the garnish. Spread out the onions on a thick layer of paper towels and cover with another thick layer. Let dry out for 30 minutes. Heat the oil in a skillet. Add the onions and cook over low heat, stirring continuously for about 20 minutes, until well browned. Add the garlic and cook, stirring continuously, for an additional 5 minutes. Remove the onions with a slotted spoon and drain well on paper towels.

4 Season the soup with salt and pepper, stir in the lemon juice and cilantro, and simmer for an additional 5 minutes. Serve garnished with the browned onions.

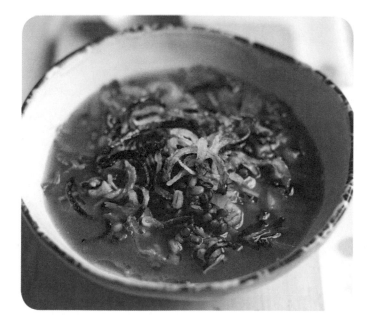

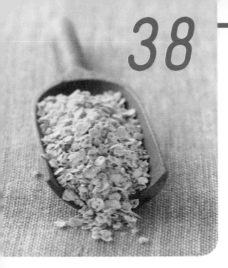

38

OATS

Economical oats are high in soluble fiber and a source of healthy fats. They can keep hunger at bay, lower bad cholesterol, and keep blood-sugar levels even.

MAJOR NUTRIENTS PER ⅓ CUP/2¼ OUNCES OATS, COOKED

Calories	233
Total fat	4g
Protein	10g
Carbohydrate	40g
Fiber	6.4g
Folate	34mcg
Vitamin B1	0.5mg
Niacin	0.6mg
Vitamin E	1.5mg
Magnesium	106mg
Potassium	257mg
Zinc	2.4g
Calcium	32mg
Iron	2.8mg

Oats have several health-giving properties. They are rich in the soluble fiber beta-glucan and have been proven to help lower bad cholesterol, boost good cholesterol, and maintain a healthy circulatory system. Oats also contain a range of antioxidants and plant chemicals to help keep heart and arteries healthy, such as avenanthramides (plant chemicals with antibiotic properties) and vitamin E. They also contain polyphenols, plant compounds that can suppress tumor growth. They are relatively low on the glycemic index (GI), which means they are a particularly useful food for dieters, people with insulin resistance, and diabetics.

• Contain plant chemicals to help reduce the risk of cancers.
• A good source of a wide range of vitamins and minerals, including the B vitamins, vitamin E, magnesium, calcium, and iron.

Practical tips:
Keep oats in an airtight container in a cool, dry, dark place and use within two to three weeks. Oat flakes can be used for making cookies and crisp toppings, and oat flour can replace wheat flour. Although oats do contain small amounts of gluten, people with gluten intolerance often find they can tolerate oats in their diet, especially if limited to no more than 1⅓ cups a day. People with a celiac condition should check with their physician before eating oats.

HONEY & OAT BARS

MAKES 16

1½ sticks unsalted butter, plus extra for greasing

3 tablespoons honey

¾ cup raw brown sugar

⅓ cup smooth peanut butter

2½ cups rolled oats

⅓ cup chopped dried apricots

2 tablespoons sunflower seeds

2 tablespoons sesame seeds

METHOD

1 Preheat the oven to 350°F. Grease and line an 8-inch square baking pan.

2 Melt the butter, honey, and sugar in a saucepan over low heat. When the butter has melted, add the peanut butter and stir until everything is well combined. Add all the remaining ingredients and mix well.

3 Press the mixture into the prepared pan and bake in the preheated oven for 20 minutes. Remove from the oven and let cool in the pan, then cut into squares and serve.

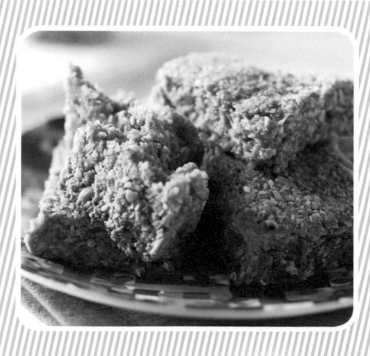

CLASSIC OATMEAL COOKIES

MAKES 30

¾ cup butter or margarine, plus extra for greasing

1⅓ cups lightly packed brown sugar

1 egg

4 tablespoons water

1 teaspoon vanilla extract

4⅓ cups rolled oats

1 cup all-purpose flour

1 teaspoon salt

⅓ teaspoon baking soda

METHOD

1 Preheat the oven to 350°F and grease a large cookie sheet.

2 Cream the butter and sugar together in a large mixing bowl. Beat in the egg, water, and vanilla extract until the mixture is smooth. In a separate bowl, mix the oats, flour, salt, and baking soda together.

3 Gradually stir the oat mixture into the butter mixture until thoroughly combined.

4 Put tablespoonfuls of the mixture onto the prepared cookie sheet, making sure they are well spaced. Transfer to the preheated oven and bake for 15 minutes, or until the cookies are golden brown.

5 Using a palette knife, carefully transfer the cookies to wire racks to cool completely.

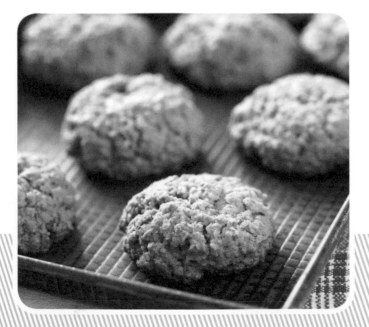

SAVORY OAT CRACKERS

MAKES 12–14

oil or melted butter,
for greasing
¾ stick plus 1 tablespoon
unsalted butter
1 cup rolled oats
¼ cup whole-wheat flour
½ teaspoon coarse sea salt
1 teaspoon dried thyme
⅓ cup finely chopped walnuts
1 egg, beaten
¼ cup sesame seeds

METHOD

1 Preheat the oven to 350°F. Lightly grease two cookie sheets.

2 Rub the butter into the oats and flour, using your fingertips. Stir in the salt, thyme, and walnuts, then add the egg and mix to a soft dough. Spread out the sesame seeds on a large shallow dish. Break off walnut-sized pieces of dough and roll into balls, then roll in the sesame seeds to coat lightly and evenly.

3 Place the balls of dough on the prepared cookie sheets, spacing well apart, and roll the rolling pin over them to flatten as much as possible. Bake in the preheated oven for 12–15 minutes, or until firm and pale golden.

4 Leave to cool on the cookie sheets for 3–4 minutes, then transfer to a wire rack to finish cooling.

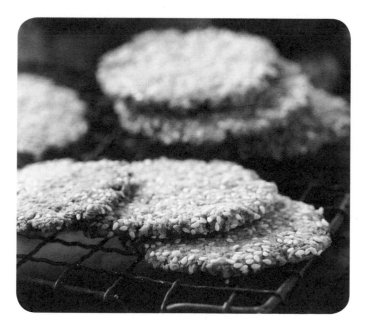

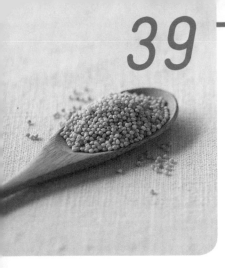

39

QUINOA

The best source of complete protein in the plant kingdom, quinoa provides all the necessary building blocks for skin, bone, and brain regeneration.

MAJOR NUTRIENTS PER ½ CUP/3½ OUNCES QUINOA, UNCOOKED

Calories	368
Total fat	6.07g
Omega-6 oils	2,977mg
Protein	14.12g
Carbohydrate	64.16g
Fiber	7mg
Vitamin B1	0.36mg
Vitamin B2	0.32mg
Vitamin B3	1.52mg
Vitamin B5	0.77mg
Vitamin B6	0.49mg
Folate	184mg
Magnesium	197mg
Iron	4.57mg
Phosphorus	457mg
Potassium	563mg
Manganese	2.03mg
Selenium	8.5mcg
Zinc	3.1mg

Most plant foods are lacking in one or more of the essential amino acids, but quinoa is an easy one-food solution, containing all the essential amino acids, plus a good range of minerals and the B vitamins. These enable the protein content of quinoa to be used effectively, so that it can provide the vast amount of energy needed for the constant renewal of skin, hair, nails, bone, and organs. Quinoa is actually a seed, not a grain. As such, it is high in anti-inflammatory omega-6 oils and is ideal for those people who cannot tolerate wheat or gluten.

• Contains phosphorus to make phospholipids in the brain and nervous system.
• Potassium balances out sodium, reducing bloating, puffiness, and high blood pressure.
• Zinc and selenium offer potent antioxidant protection.

Practical tips:
Stored correctly, quinoa will last for up to a year in an airtight container. Keep in a cool, dry, dark place for best results. Cook quinoa in a similar way to rice. It has a pleasant, nutty flavor, and is delicious in Mexican and Indian meals. You can also make a great hot quinoa, either from flakes or from the grain itself. Quinoa is versatile enough to be cooked in both sweet desserts and unsweetened dishes.

TABBOULEH

SERVES 4

1½ cups quinoa

2½ cups water

10 vine-ripened cherry tomatoes, halved

3-inch piece cucumber, quartered and sliced

3 scallions, finely chopped

juice of ½ lemon

2 tablespoons extra virgin olive oil

¼ cup chopped fresh mint

¼ cup chopped fresh cilantro

¼ cup chopped fresh parsley

salt and pepper, to taste

METHOD

1 Put the quinoa into a medium saucepan and cover with the water. Bring to a boil, then reduce the heat, cover, and simmer over low heat for 15 minutes. Drain if necessary.

2 Let the quinoa cool slightly before combining with the remaining ingredients in a salad bowl. Adjust the seasoning, if necessary, before serving.

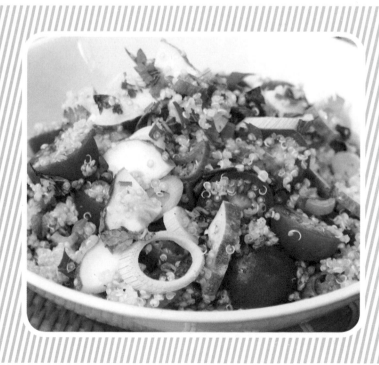

CHICKPEA & QUINOA SALAD

SERVES 4

⅓ cup red quinoa
1 red chile, seeded and finely chopped
8 scallions, chopped
3 tablespoons finely chopped fresh mint
2 tablespoons olive oil
2 tablespoons fresh lemon juice
⅓ cup chickpea (besan) flour
1 teaspoon ground cumin
½ teaspoon paprika
1 tablespoon vegetable oil
1 cup drained and rinsed, canned chickpeas

METHOD

1   Put the quinoa in a medium saucepan and cover with boiling water. Place over low heat and simmer for 10 minutes, or until just cooked. Drain and refresh with cold water, drain again. Transfer to a large bowl and toss together with the red chile, scallions, and mint to mix thoroughly.

2   Combine the olive oil and lemon juice in a small bowl, using a fork.

3   Sift together the chickpea flour, cumin, and paprika into a wide, deep bowl. Put the vegetable oil in a medium skillet over medium heat. Roll the chickpeas in the spiced flour, then cook gently in the skillet, stirring frequently, for 2–3 minutes, letting the chickpeas brown in patches.

4   Stir the warm chickpeas into the quinoa mixture and quickly stir in the lemon-oil dressing. Serve warm or chilled.

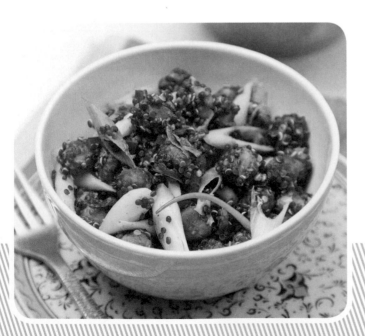

QUINOA WITH ROASTED VEGETABLES

SERVES 2–4

2 bell peppers (any color), seeded and cut into chunky pieces

1 large zucchini, cut into chunks

1 small fennel bulb, cut into slim wedges

1 tablespoon olive oil

2 teaspoons finely chopped fresh rosemary leaves

1 teaspoon chopped fresh thyme leaves

generous ½ cup quinoa

1½ cups vegetable stock

2 garlic cloves, peeled and crushed

3 tablespoons chopped fresh flat-leaf parsley

⅓ cup pine nuts, toasted

salt and pepper, to taste

METHOD

1 Preheat the oven to 400°F. Put the bell peppers, zucchini, and fennel in a roasting pan large enough to hold the vegetables in a single layer.

2 Drizzle the olive oil over the vegetables and sprinkle with the rosemary and thyme. Season well with salt and pepper, then mix well with clean hands. Roast for 25–30 minutes, until tender and lightly charred.

3 Meanwhile, put the quinoa, stock, and garlic in a pan. Bring to a boil, cover, and simmer for 12–15 minutes, until tender and most of the stock has been absorbed.

4 Remove the vegetables from the oven. Turn the quinoa into the roasting pan. Add the parsley and pine nuts, and toss together. Serve warm or cold.

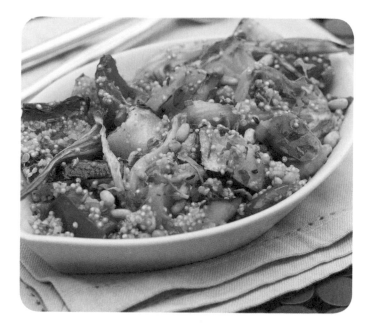

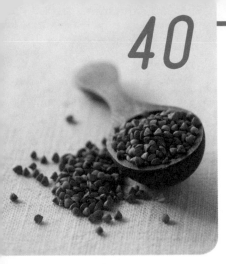

40

BUCKWHEAT

Buckwheat contains a rich supply of flavonoids, particularly rutin. These help to keep blood circulation flowing freely and prevent varicose veins.

Buckwheat is technically a seed, not a grain, so it is an excellent source of fiber and energy for people who are intolerant to wheat and gluten. Whether you have an intolerance or not, reducing your wheat intake could be beneficial—buckwheat is easier to digest than wheat and also more alkalizing, meaning that it helps the body's physical processes work more efficiently. It is a particularly sustaining energy source and is recommended for diabetics, because it releases its sugars slowly into the bloodstream. Buckwheat, like millet, also contains substances called nutrilosides that are essential in detoxification processes, helping rid the body of harmful, aging toxins.

- Contains lecithin, which helps break down fats in the liver and in the food that you eat, aiding detoxification and reducing cravings for fatty foods.
- Magnesium and potassium work together to ensure a healthy heart and strong bones.
- Selenium produces both of the rejuvenating antioxidants glutathione and coenzyme Q-10.

Practical tips:
Buckwheat may be used as an alternative to rice. It can also be bought in flakes and served as a hot breakfast cereal. Buckwheat flour makes excellent gluten-free pancakes, which are traditional in Poland and Russia, and also eaten in France.

MAJOR NUTRIENTS PER ½ CUP/3½ OUNCES BUCKWHEAT, UNCOOKED

Calories	343
Total fat	3.4g
Omega-6 oils	1,052mg
Protein	13.25g
Carbohydrate	71.5g
Fiber	10mg
Vitamin B2	0.43mg
Vitamin B3	7.02mg
Vitamin B5	1.23mg
Vitamin B6	0.21mg
Folate	30mcg
Magnesium	231mg
Potassium	460mg
Manganese	1.33mg
Selenium	8.3mcg
Zinc	2.4mcg

RAW BUCKWHEAT & ALMOND OATMEAL

SERVES 6

½ cup whole blanched almonds, soaked overnight in water

1¼ cups water

OATMEAL

2 cups raw buckwheat groats, soaked in cold water for 90 minutes

1 teaspoon cinnamon

2 tablespoons light agave nectar, plus extra to serve

sliced strawberries, to serve

METHOD

1   To make the almond milk, drain the almonds and transfer to a blender or food processor. Blend the almonds with the water. Keep the blender running for a minute or two to break down the almonds as much as possible.

2   Pour the mixture into a strainer lined with cheesecloth and squeeze through as much of the liquid as possible into a large bowl or liquid measuring cup. You should get approximately 1¼ cups of raw almond milk.

3   Rinse the soaked buckwheat thoroughly in cold water. Transfer to the blender or food processor with the almond milk, cinnamon, and agave nectar. Blend to a slightly coarse texture.

4   Chill the mixture for at least 30 minutes or overnight. It can be stored, covered, in the refrigerator for 3 days.

5   Serve in small bowls, topped with strawberries and extra agave nectar.

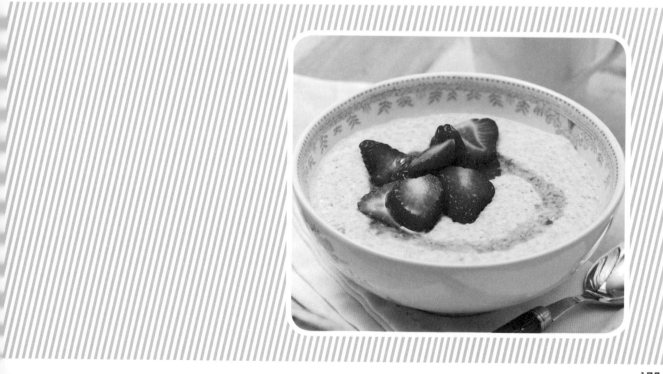

BUCKWHEAT, FETA & TOMATO SALAD

SERVES 4

2 tablespoons olive oil

1 onion, chopped

2 garlic cloves, crushed

1 cup buckwheat groats

1 (14½-ounce) can diced tomatoes

½ teaspoon tomato paste

1 cup low-sodium vegetable stock

1 tablespoon chopped fresh sage, or 1 teaspoon dried sage

pinch of crushed red pepper

¾ cup crumbled, drained feta cheese

salt and pepper

METHOD

1 Heat the oil in a deep skillet with a tight-fitting lid over medium–high heat. Add the onion and garlic and sauté for 5 minutes. Add the buckwheat and sauté for an additional 1 minute.

2 Add the tomatoes with their can juices, the tomato paste, stock, sage, and crushed red pepper and season with salt and pepper. Bring to a boil, stirring continuously, then reduce the heat to low, cover the pan, and let simmer for 20–25 minutes, or until the liquid has been absorbed and the buckwheat is tender.

3 Lightly stir in the feta cheese, replace the lid, and let the buckwheat stand for up to 20 minutes. Just before serving, lightly stir with a fork.

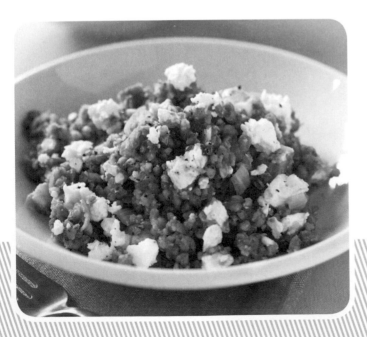

BUCKWHEAT SODA BREAD

MAKES 1 LOAF

1 cup buckwheat flour, plus extra for sprinkling

⅔ cup rice flour

1 teaspoon salt

1 teaspoon xanthan gum

2 teaspoons gluten-free baking powder

1¼ cups milk, plus extra for glazing

1 teaspoon white wine vinegar

1 tablespoon olive oil

METHOD

1   Preheat the oven to 400°F. Sift together the buckwheat flour, rice flour, salt, xanthan gum, and baking powder into a bowl and make a well in the center.

2   Mix together the milk, vinegar, and oil and stir into the dry ingredients to make a soft dough.

3   Sprinkle a little flour over a baking sheet. Shape the dough into a smooth 8-inch circle and place on the baking sheet. Lightly press to flatten, then use a sharp knife to cut a deep cross into the loaf.

4   Brush with milk to glaze and bake in the preheated oven for 25–30 minutes, or until risen, firm, and golden brown. Transfer to a wire rack to cool.

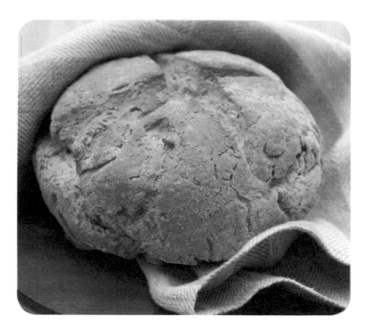

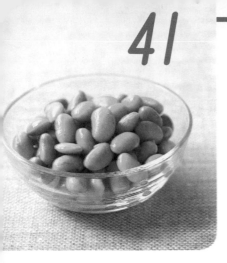

41

MISO

Miso is a traditional Japanese ingredient used as a seasoning in dishes—the Japanese diet has long been associated with long life and good health.

MAJOR NUTRIENTS PER 1 TABLESPOON MISO

Calories	34
Total fat	1.03g
Protein	2.01g
Carbohydrate	4.55g
Fiber	0.93g
Vitamin B1	0.02mg
Vitamin B2	0.04mg
Vitamin B3	0.16mg
Vitamin B5	0.06mg
Vitamin B6	0.03mg
Vitamin B12	0.43mcg
Vitamin K	8.53mcg
Iron	0.43mg
Selenium	1.2mcg
Zinc	0.44mg
Manganese	0.3mg

Miso is a traditional Japanese seasoning, most often produced by fermenting soybeans with salt and koji yeast mold, although it can also be made with rice, wheat, or barley. Like yogurt and kefir, miso is associated with good digestive health, because it feeds the beneficial probiotic bacteria present in the body. This supports toxin elimination and the absorption of nutrients to keep the body healthy. Fermented foods also help the immune system, helping to reduce multiple sensitivities and inflammation, as seen in hay fever and skin problems.

- Contains tryptophan, needed for serotonin production, which encourages good mood and restorative sleep.
- Manganese makes the detoxifying antioxidant enzyme superoxide dismutase.
- Vitamin K transports calcium around the body in support of good bone health and efficient blood clotting.
- Zinc-rich food that promotes optimal immune function and rapid healing, helping your skin look more youthful.

Practical tips:
Miso is salty, but a little goes a long way in terms of taste and mineral content. The paste is superior to the powdered form and can be used to make an instant, simple soup when mixed with boiling water. Add miso to boiled vegetables and ginger to make a heartier broth, which you can supplement with shrimp, chicken, or tofu.

MISO SOUP

SERVES 4

4 cups water

2 teaspoons dashi granules

¾ cup diced, drained silken tofu

4 shiitake mushrooms, finely sliced

¼ cup miso paste

2 scallions, chopped

METHOD

1   Put the water in a large saucepan with the dashi granules and bring to a boil. Add the tofu and mushrooms, reduce the heat, and let simmer for 3 minutes.

2   Stir in the miso paste and let simmer gently, stirring, until the miso has dissolved.

3   Add the scallions and serve immediately. If you let the soup stand, the miso will settle, so stir before serving to recombine.

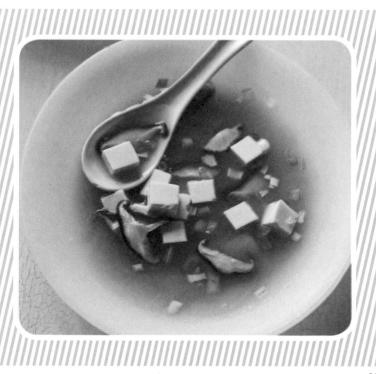

QUICK GINGER & MISO STIR-FRY

SERVES 2

1 teaspoon miso paste

1 tablespoon tomato paste

1-inch piece fresh ginger, peeled

3 tablespoons vegetable oil

1 green bell pepper, seeded and thinly sliced

1 red bell pepper, seeded and thinly sliced

¼ green cabbage, cored and thinly sliced

1 carrot, thinly sliced

1 red chile, seeded and finely chopped

6 scallions, finely chopped

⅓ cup edamame (green soybeans)

⅓ cup coarsely chopped cashew nuts

cooked rice, to serve

METHOD

1 To make the sauce, dissolve the miso paste in 2 tablespoons of boiling water. Mix together the warm miso and the tomato paste in a small bowl. Grate the ginger coarsely, then gather up the grated ginger and squeeze the juice into the miso mixture.

2 Heat the vegetable oil in a large wok over high heat. Stir-fry the bell peppers, cabbage, carrot, chile, scallions, edamame, and nuts for 5 minutes.

3 Stir in the miso-ginger sauce and cook for an additional minute.

4 Serve immediately, with cooked rice.

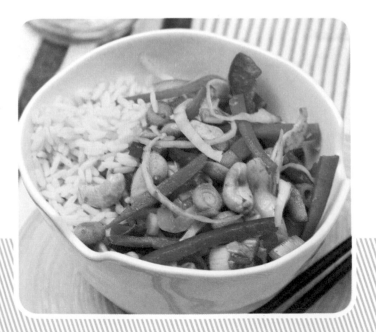

BEEF & MISO STIR-FRY

SERVES 3

2 rump steaks, weighing
1 pound in total

8 tablespoons store-bought
miso glaze

4 tablespoons groundnut oil

2 shallots, chopped

1 large garlic clove,
finely chopped

1-inch piece fresh ginger,
finely chopped

2 carrots, finely sliced

½ green hispi cabbage,
halved lengthways and
cored, leaves sliced
crossways

3 tablespoons chicken stock

5½ ounces enoki mushrooms,
base removed

2 tablespoons sesame seeds

small handful coriander
leaves, roughly chopped

METHOD

1 Put the steaks between two sheets of plastic wrap and pound with a meat mallet to a thickness of ¼ inch. Slice into 2-inch x 1-inch strips. Put into a shallow dish and stir in the miso glaze. Cover and leave to marinate in the refrigerator overnight.

2 Drain the beef, reserving the excess marinade.

3 Heat a large wok over a high heat. Add half the groundnut oil and heat until very hot. Add the beef and stir-fry for 3 minutes until brown. Remove from the wok and keep warm.

4 Wipe the wok with kitchen paper. Heat over medium heat, add the remaining oil and heat until hot. Add the shallots and stir-fry for 2 minutes, then add the garlic and ginger and cook for 15 seconds.

5 Stir in the carrots and cabbage. Increase the heat to medium–high and stir in the stock and reserved marinade. Stir-fry for 3 minutes, until tender. Break up the mushrooms, add to the wok and stir-fry for 30 seconds.

6 Return the meat to the wok and stir-fry for 1 minute, or until heated through. Sprinkle over sesame seeds and coriander and serve immediately.

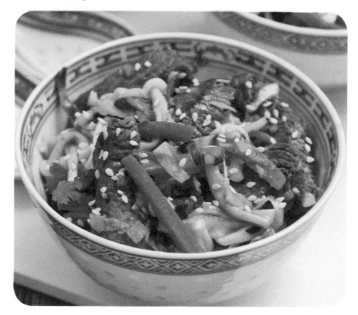

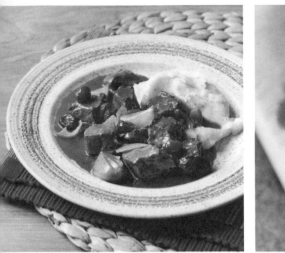

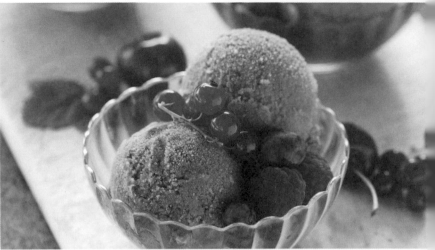

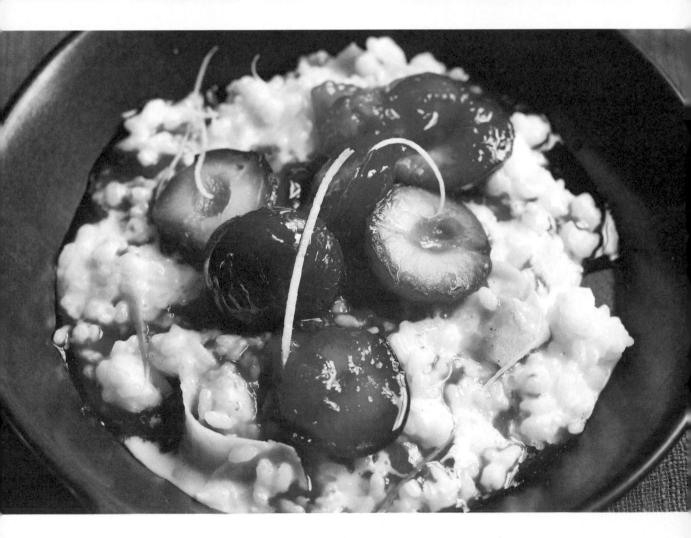

HERBS & FLAVORINGS

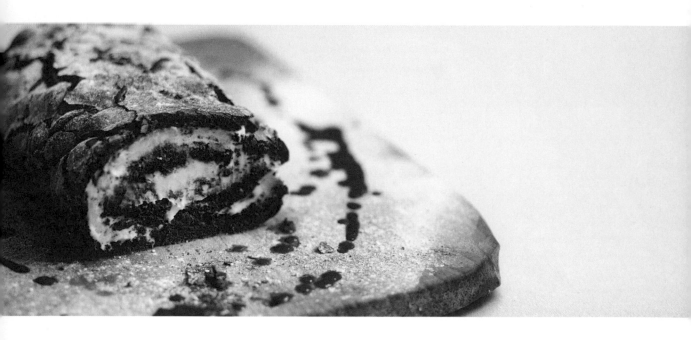

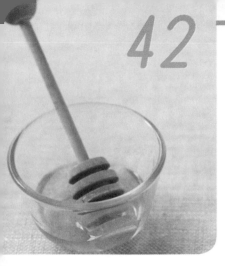

42

HONEY

Raw honey is one of nature's oldest known antibacterial products. Used topically, honey has an antiseptic and antibacterial effect.

MAJOR NUTRIENTS PER 1 TABLESPOON HONEY

Calories	45.5
Total fat	0g
Protein	0.04g
Carbohydrate	12.36g
Fiber	0.03g

Honey is created when the saliva of bees meets the nectar they collect from flowers, so the properties of a particular honey will reflect those of the flowers the bees have visited most prominently. In its raw state, it contains an array of antioxidants, such as chrysin and vitamin C, but these properties are destroyed when it is excessively heated or processed. Manuka honey from New Zealand is the only honey that has been tested for its ability to destroy harmful bacteria, and batches of this are given a Unique Manuka Factor (UMF) according to strength. Manuka has been shown to be twice as effective as other honeys against *E. coli* and *Staphylococcus* bacteria, which commonly infect wounds.

- Raw honey contains propolis, which helps reduce inflammation and premature aging.
- Good-quality honey contains probiotic benefical bacteria lactobacilli and bifidobacteria to support immunity.
- When applied to the skin, it has been shown to help heal pimples, burns, cuts, and sores.

Practical tips:
Choose good-quality honey—look for local, raw, and unprocessed varieties from farm shops. Darker types, such as buckwheat and sage, contain the most antioxidants, and the honey produced by flower-fed bees in the summer contains more beneficial bacteria.

DID YOU KNOW?

When mixed with water, honey creates antiseptic hydrogen peroxide, which can be applied directly to wounds to dry them out and keep them free from infection while they heal.

HONEY & LEMON MUFFINS

MAKES 12

1 cup gluten-free, wheat-free all-purpose flour

¾ cup plus 2 tablespoons cornmeal

¼ cup granulated sugar

2 teaspoons gluten-free baking powder

¼ teaspoon xanthan gum

1 egg

juice and zest of ⅓ lemon

¼ cup vegetable oil

1 cup milk

2 tablespoons honey

1 tablespoon glycerin

METHOD

1   Preheat the oven to 350°F. Line a 12-cup muffin pan with muffin cups.

2   Put the flour, cornmeal, sugar, baking powder, and xanthan gum into a bowl and mix together well.

3   In a separate bowl, mix together all the remaining liquid ingredients. Add the liquid mixture to the dry mixture and fold in gently.

4   Spoon the batter into the muffin cups and bake the muffins in the preheated oven for 18–20 minutes, until well risen and golden. Remove from the oven and cool on a wire rack.

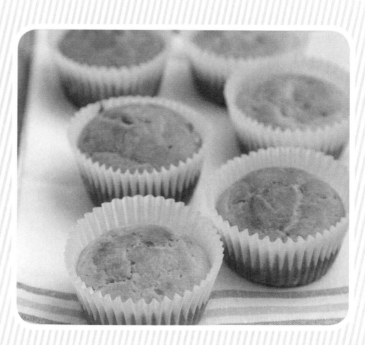

HONEY & PISTACHIO ICE CREAM

SERVES 10

6 egg yolks
2 teaspoons cornstarch
⅓ cup honey
2 cups milk
1 cup Greek yogurt
2 teaspoons rosewater
(optional)
½ cup coarsely chopped
pistachio nuts
poached figs, to serve

METHOD

1   Put the egg yolks, cornstarch, and honey into a large mixing bowl. Put the milk into a medium, heavy saucepan, bring to a boil, then gradually whisk it into the yolks. Strain the mixture through a strainer back into the pan and cook over low heat, stirring, until thickened and smooth. Pour the custard into a clean bowl, cover the surface with plastic wrap, and let cool.

2   Whisk the yogurt and rosewater, if using, into the custard. Pour the mixture into a chilled ice-cream machine and churn for 15–20 minutes, until thick and creamy. Mix in the pistachio nuts and churn until stiff enough to scoop. If you don't have an ice-cream machine, pour into a large nonstick loaf pan for 3–4 hours, until semifrozen. Beat in a food processor, then stir in the pistachio nuts, return to the loaf pan, and freeze for an additional 3 hours, or until firm.

3   When ready to serve, take the ice cream out of the freezer and let it soften at room temperature for 5–10 minutes. Scoop into small dishes and add 2 fig halves. Serve immediately.

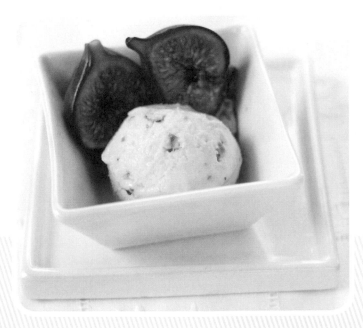

HONEY & MUSTARD CHICKEN PASTA SALAD

SERVES 4

8 ounces dried fusilli

2 tablespoons olive oil

1 onion, thinly sliced

1 garlic clove, crushed

4 skinless, boneless chicken breasts (about 4 ounces each), thinly sliced

2 tablespoons whole-grain mustard

2 tablespoons honey

10 cherry tomatoes, halved

handful of mizuna or arugula leaves

fresh thyme leaves, to garnish

DRESSING

3 tablespoons olive oil

1 tablespoon sherry vinegar

2 teaspoons honey

1 tablespoon fresh thyme leaves

salt and pepper

METHOD

1 To make the dressing, put all the ingredients, including salt and pepper to taste, in a small bowl and whisk together until well blended.

2 Bring a large, heavy saucepan of lightly salted water to a boil. Add the fusilli, bring back to a boil, and cook according to the package directions, until just tender but still firm to the bite.

3 Meanwhile, heat the oil in a large skillet. Add the onion and garlic and sauté for 5 minutes. Add the chicken and cook, stirring frequently, for 3–4 minutes. Stir the mustard and honey into the skillet and cook for an additional 2–3 minutes, until the chicken and onion are golden brown and sticky. Check that the chicken is tender and cooked through—when cut through with a knife, there should be no signs of pinkness.

4 Drain the pasta and transfer to a serving bowl. Pour the dressing over the pasta and toss well. Stir in the chicken and onion and let cool.

5 Gently stir the tomatoes and mizuna into the pasta. Serve garnished with thyme leaves.

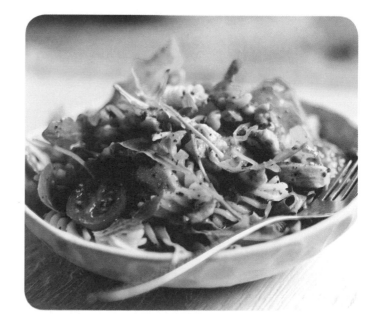

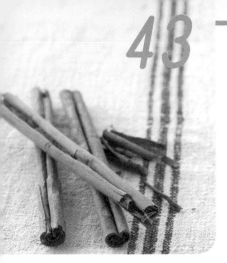

43

CINNAMON

Cinnamon is an anti-inflammatory, antibacterial spice that can help relieve bloating and heartburn, and it offers protection against strokes.

**MAJOR NUTRIENTS PER
2 TABLESPOONS/½ OUNCE
CINNAMON**

Calories	18
Total fat	Trace
Protein	Trace
Carbohydrate	5.5g
Fiber	3.7g
Folate	287mcg
Potassium	34mg
Calcium	84mg
Iron	2.6mg

Cinnamon contains several oils and compounds, including cinnamaldehyde, cinnamyl acetate, and cinnamyl alcohol, which have a variety of beneficial actions. Cinnamaldehyde has an anticoagulant action, meaning that it can help to protect against strokes, and is also anti-inflammatory, relieving symptoms of arthritis and asthma. The spice is a digestive aid, relieving bloating and flatulence, and it can reduce the discomfort of heartburn. Cinnamon has antibacterial action that can block the yeast fungus candida and bugs that can cause food poisoning. In one study, cinnamon was shown to lower blood sugar and blood cholesterol.

• Helps to combat indigestion and bloating.
• Antibacterial and antifungal.
• Helps prevent blood clots.
• May lower bad cholesterol and blood sugar.

Practical tips:
True cinnamon is the inner bark of an evergreen tree of the laurel family native to Sri Lanka, and cassia is another variety native to China. Both are widely available, but it is not always possible to know which one you are buying. Whole bark cinnamon sticks will retain their flavor and aroma for up to a year, while the ground dried spice will last for about six months. Whole or pieces of cinammon sticks and ground cinnamon, can be used to flavor both sweet and unsweetened dishes.

CINNAMON & WALNUT LAYER CAKE

SERVES 10

1 cup firmly packed
light brown sugar
2 cups all-purpose flour
2 teaspoons ground cinnamon
1 teaspoon baking soda
3 eggs, beaten
1 cup sunflower oil,
plus extra for greasing
1 cup finely chopped walnuts
1 large ripe banana, mashed
walnut pieces, to decorate

FROSTING
¾ cup cream cheese
2 sticks unsalted butter
1 teaspoon ground cinnamon
1¾ cups confectioners' sugar

METHOD

1 Preheat the oven to 350°F. Grease three 8-inch cake pans and line with parchment paper.

2 Put the brown sugar into a large bowl and sift in the flour, cinnamon, and baking soda. Add the eggs, oil, walnuts, and banana and beat with a wooden spoon until thoroughly mixed.

3 Divide the batter among the prepared pans and gently smooth the surfaces. Bake in the preheated oven for 20–25 minutes, or until golden brown and firm to the touch. Let cool in the pans for 10 minutes, then invert onto a wire rack to cool completely.

4 To make the frosting, put the cream cheese, butter, and cinnamon into a bowl and beat together until smooth and creamy. Stir in the confectioners' sugar and mix until smooth.

5 Sandwich together the three cakes with one-third of the frosting and spread the remainder over the top and sides of the cake. Decorate with the walnut pieces.

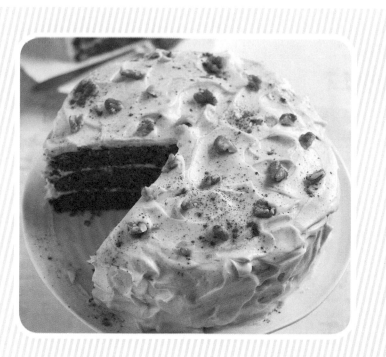

CINNAMON COFFEE ROLLS

MAKES 9

3¼ cups white bread flour, plus extra for dusting

¼ teaspoon salt

1½ teaspoons active dry yeast

¼ cup granulated sugar

4 tablespoons butter, melted, plus extra for greasing

1 egg, beaten

1 cup lukewarm milk

oil, for greasing

3 tablespoons butter, softened

¼ cup firmly packed dark brown sugar

1½ teaspoons instant coffee powder

1 teaspoon ground cinnamon

1 cup confectioners' sugar, mixed with 1 tablespoon water, to decorate

METHOD

1 Sift the flour and salt into a large bowl. Stir in the yeast and sugar and make a well in the center. Beat together the melted butter, egg, and milk, then pour into the well and mix to a dough. Turn out the dough onto a lightly floured surface and knead for 5–6 minutes, until smooth and elastic. Place the dough in a bowl, cover with lightly oiled plastic wrap, and let rest in a warm place for 1½ hours, or until doubled in size. Grease a 9-inch square cake pan.

2 Turn out the dough onto a floured surface and lightly knead for 1 minute. Roll out to a 12-inch square. Spread the butter over the dough. Mix together the sugar, coffee, and cinnamon and sprinkle over the butter in an even layer. Roll up the dough from one side, then cut into nine circles and place cut-side up in the prepared pan. Cover loosely with oiled plastic wrap and let rest for 40–50 minutes, or until doubled in size. Meanwhile, preheat the oven to 400°F.

3 Bake the rolls in the preheated oven for 18–20 minutes, or until risen and golden. Invert onto a wire rack to cool completely. Drizzle the icing over the rolls, let set, then pull apart to serve.

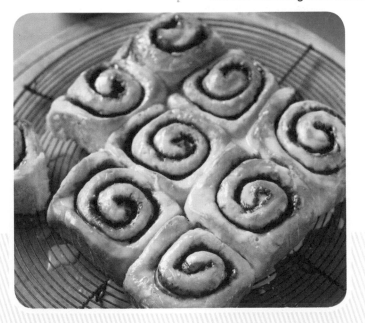

RICE PUDDING WITH CINNAMON-POACHED PLUMS

SERVES 4

½ cup short-grain rice

2 tablespoons sugar

1 tablespoon unsalted butter

2 cups milk

thinly pared strip of orange rind

shreds of orange zest, to decorate

COMPOTE

8 red plums, halved and pitted

1 cinnamon stick

2 tablespoons sugar

juice of 1 orange

METHOD

1 Put the rice, sugar, and butter into a saucepan and stir in the milk and orange rind. Heat gently, stirring occasionally, until almost boiling.

2 Reduce the heat to low, then cover and simmer gently for 40–45 minutes, stirring occasionally, until the rice is tender and most of the liquid has been absorbed.

3 Meanwhile, to make the compote, put the plums, cinnamon, sugar, and orange juice into a large saucepan. Heat gently until just boiling, then reduce the heat, cover, and simmer gently for about 10 minutes, or until the plums are tender.

4 Remove the plums with a slotted spoon and discard the cinnamon. Serve the rice pudding warm with the compote and sprinkled with orange zest.

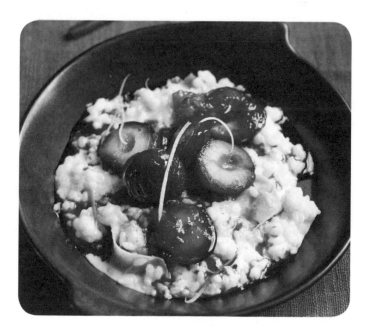

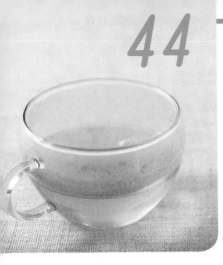

44

GREEN TEA

The Chinese and Japanese have long understood the health attributes of green tea, and they view it as an important way to care for their heart, energy, and skin.

MAJOR NUTRIENTS PER 1 CUP GREEN TEA

Calories	2
Total fat	0g
Protein	0g
Carbohydrate	Trace
Fiber	0g
Catechins	3.75g

The leaves of the tea plant *Camellia sinensis* are loaded with catechins, which have been found to have natural antioxidant, antibacterial, and antiviral properties, thereby protecting against cancer and helping to lower cholesterol and regulate blood clotting. One such compound, epigallocatechin gallate (EGCG), is able to penetrate the cells and protect the crucial DNA that the body relies on to replicate cells and combat the damage caused by aging. EGCG also prevents cancer cells from forming and can help reduce the severity of allergies by blocking the body's response.

- May act as a weight-loss aid by helping to burn fat and regulate blood-sugar and insulin levels.
- Contains quercetin, a bioflavonoid (plant chemical) that reduces inflammation and helps control food allergies.
- Catechins promote liver detoxification, thus assisting in the removal of aging toxins and promoting glowing skin.

Practical tips:
Changing from black tea or coffee to green tea will lower your intake of caffeine and its aging effects. Green tea leaves are the dried leaves of the tea plant, while black, "normal" tea is fermented. The fermentation process makes black tea much higher in caffeine: about 50 mg a cup compared with 5 mg for green tea. Different varieties have different strengths and taste, so it's advisable to experiment to find the one you enjoy most.

GREEN TEA & YELLOW PLUM SMOOTHIE

SERVES 2

1 green tea bag

1¼ cups boiling water

1 teaspoon good-quality honey, or to taste (optional)

2 ripe yellow plums, halved and pitted

METHOD

1   Put the tea bag in a teapot or heatproof bowl and pour over the boiling water. Let steep for 7 minutes. Remove and discard the tea bag. Let cool, then chill in the refrigerator.

2   Pour the chilled tea into a food processor or blender. Add the honey, if using, and plums, and process until smooth.

3   Serve at once.

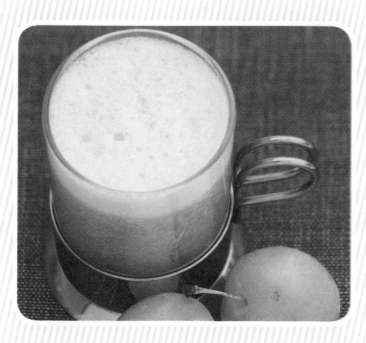

EN TEA & HAZELNUT CREAM

SERVES 6

1¾ cups canned coconut milk

2½ cups fresh finely grated coconut

1 cup superfine sugar or granulated sugar

1 tablespoon green tea (matcha) powder

½ cup roasted hazelnuts, chopped

METHOD

1 Put the coconut milk and grated coconut in a medium saucepan over medium heat and mix together.

2 Whisk in the sugar and green tea powder and heat until the sugar has dissolved. Stir in the chopped hazelnuts and set aside to cool to room temperature.

3 Transfer to an ice-cream maker and churn according to the manufacturer's directions. Alternatively, pour the cooled mixture into a shallow freezerproof container and place in the freezer. Let freeze until not quite set, then remove from the freezer, beat, and freeze again until firm. Store in the freezer until required.

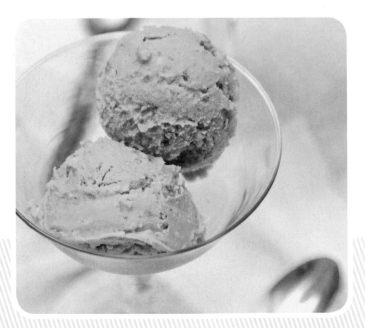

GREEN TEA & POMEGRANATE CUPCAKES

MAKES 12

1½ cups all-purpose flour

1½ teaspoons baking powder

1 tablespoon green tea (matcha) powder

¼ teaspoon salt

1 stick unsalted butter, softened

1 cup superfine sugar or granulated sugar

1 teaspoon vanilla extract

2 eggs

½ cup pomegranate syrup

4 tablespoons milk

FROSTING

1 stick unsalted butter, softened

1½–2 cups confectioners' sugar (see method)

¼ cup pomegranate seeds, to decorate

METHOD

1 Preheat the oven to 350°F. Line a 12-cup cupcake pan with paper liners.

2 Sift together the flour, baking powder, green tea powder, and salt in a bowl. Put the butter and superfine sugar into a separate bowl and beat until pale and fluffy. Add the vanilla extract, and the eggs. Add half of the flour mixture, ¼ cup of the pomegranate syrup, and the milk and mix to incorporate. Add the remaining flour mixture and mix.

3 Spoon the batter into the paper liners and bake in the preheated oven for 20 minutes, or until a toothpick inserted into the center of a cupcake comes out clean. Let cool in the pan for 1–2 minutes, then transfer to a wire rack to cool completely.

4 To make the frosting, put the butter, 1½ cups confectioners' sugar, and the remaining pomegranate syrup in a bowl and beat with an electric mixer until well combined. Add more confectioners' sugar, if necessary, to achieve a piping consistency. Spoon the frosting into a pastry bag fitted with a star-shaped tip and pipe onto the cupcakes. Sprinkle with pomegranate seeds and serve.

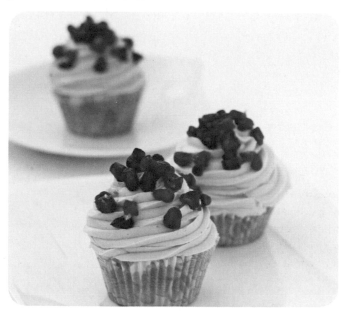

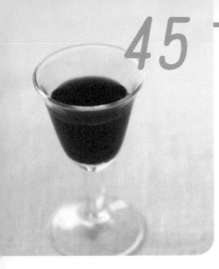

45

RED WINE

Red wine is an important contributor to the age-defying Mediterranean diet. Enjoyed in moderation, it offers excellent heart-protecting properties.

The high antioxidant action of red wine comes from a substance called resveratrol, which is found in red grape skins in much higher amounts than in any other food. The major action of resveratrol means that drinking red wine regularly in moderation—less than 5 fluid ounces a day—can make blood platelets less sticky and help blood vessels stay open and flexible. These are both important considerations in regulating blood pressure and, therefore, cutting the risk of heart disease. Drinking red wine has been estimated to add a year to life expectancy, especially if only drunk with food and alongside a healthy diet.

- Resveratrol is an effective agent in disease prevention.
- It has also been shown to have a potent anti-inflammatory action, supporting healthy skin and trouble-free joints.
- Cabernet Sauvignon, in particular, has been shown to help improve the memory deterioration shown in Alzheimer's disease.

Practical tips:
Straying above the recommended one glass a day for women and two glasses a day for men soon negates the benefits of red wine. Quality is also key: the deeper the red, the higher the antioxidant count. The greatest amounts are found in Merlot, Cabernet Sauvignon, and Sangiovese grapes. Rioja and Pinot Noir offer moderate amounts, while the least benefit is derived from Côtes du Rhône.

MAJOR NUTRIENTS PER ½ CUP RED WINE

Calories	95
Total fat	0g
Protein	0.07g
Carbohydrate	2.87g
Fiber	Trace
Vitamin C	Trace
Potassium	Trace
Lycopene	Trace
Lutein/Zeaxanthin	145.6mg

DID YOU KNOW?

Sipping red wine slowly may increase the blood levels of resveratrol by 100 times, because it is absorbed much better through the mouth than the digestive tract.

RED WINE BRAISED CABBAGE

SERVES 6

2 tablespoons butter

1 garlic clove, chopped

1 head red cabbage, shredded

1 cup golden raisins

1 tablespoon good-quality honey

½ cup red wine

½ cup water

METHOD

1 Melt the butter in a large saucepan over medium heat. Add the garlic and cook, stirring, for 1 minute, until slightly softened.

2 Add the cabbage and golden raisins, then stir in the honey. Cook for an additional 1 minute.

3 Pour in the wine and water and bring to a boil. Reduce the heat, cover, and simmer gently, stirring occasionally, for 45 minutes, or until the cabbage is cooked. Serve hot.

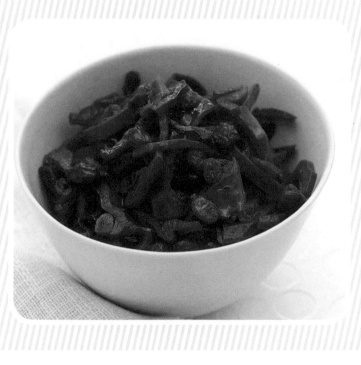

BRAISED BEEF WITH RED WINE & CRANBERRIES

SERVES 4

2 tablespoons olive oil

6 shallots, quartered

1¼ pounds chuck steak, cubed

1 tablespoon all-purpose flour

1¼ cups red wine

2 tablespoons tomato paste

1 tablespoon Worcestershire sauce

2 bay leaves

1 cup fresh or frozen cranberries

salt and pepper

mashed potatoes and seasonal vegetables, to serve

METHOD

1 Heat the oil in a large, flameproof casserole dish, add the shallots, and sauté, stirring, for 2–3 minutes, until beginning to brown. Remove from the dish and keep warm.

2 Add the steak and cook, stirring, for 3–4 minutes, or until evenly browned. Stir in the flour and cook for 1 minute.

3 Add the wine and bring to a boil, then boil for 1 minute. Return the shallots to the dish with the tomato paste, Worcestershire sauce, and bay leaves and season with salt and pepper. Stir in the cranberries.

4 Reduce the heat to low, cover tightly with a lid, and let simmer gently for 1–1½ hours, until the beef is tender.

5 Remove and discard the bay leaves, adjust the seasoning, if desired, and serve with mashed potatoes and vegetables.

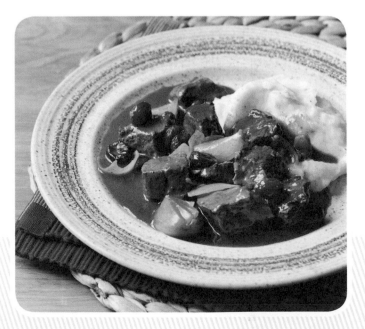

RED WINE SORBET

MAKES 6

1 orange

1 lemon

2½ cups fruity red wine

½ cup lightly packed soft brown sugar

1¼ cups water, chilled

2 large egg whites, lightly beaten

redcurrants, blueberries, cherries and raspberries, to serve

METHOD

1 Peel the zest from the orange and lemon in strips using a potato peeler, being careful not to remove any of the bitter white pith underneath. Put in a saucepan with the red wine and sugar. Heat gently, stirring until the sugar dissolves, then bring to a boil and simmer for 5 minutes. Remove from the heat and stir in the water.

2 Squeeze the juice from the fruit. Stir into the wine mixture. Cover and leave until completely cooled, then strain into a freezerproof container. Cover and freeze for 7–8 hours, or until firm.

3 Working quickly, break the sorbet into chunks and transfer to a food processor. Blend for a few seconds to break down the chunks, then, leaving the processor running, gradually pour the egg whites through the feed tube. The mixture will become paler. Continue blending until smooth.

4 Freeze for a further 3–4 hours, or until firm. Scoop into six chilled glasses and serve immediately with redcurrants, blueberries, cherries and raspberries.

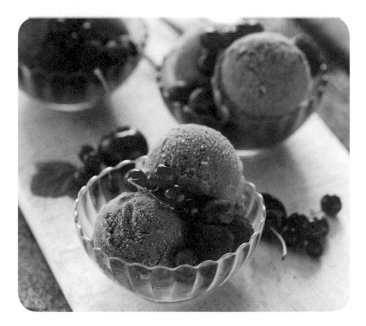

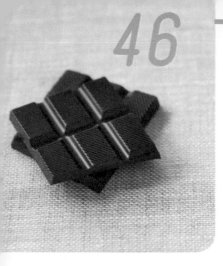

46

DARK CHOCOLATE

Our love affair with chocolate is rooted in its health-giving properties. The cacao bean is loaded with nutrients, mood-enhancing chemicals, and antioxidants.

MAJOR NUTRIENTS PER 3½ OUNCES DARK CHOCOLATE (70–85 PERCENT COCOA SOLIDS)

Calories	598
Total fat	42.63g
Omega-9 oils	12,652mg
Protein	7.79g
Carbohydrate	45.9g
Fiber	10.9g
Vitamin B3	1.05mg
Vitamin B5	0.42mg
Magnesium	228mg
Potassium	716mg
Phosphorus	308mg
Iron	11.9mg
Manganese	1.95mg
Selenium	6.8mcg
Zinc	3.31mg
Caffeine	75.6mg
Theobromine	448.8mg

The bean from which we make our favorite confectionery is highly nutritious; it's packed full of rejuvenating potassium, magnesium, vitamins B3 and B5, zinc, and selenium. However, its true potency comes from its high antioxidant content. Chocolate contains more than four times the catechins present in green tea and twice as much as in red wine. These substances lower the risk of both heart attacks and cancer by reducing inflammation and helping renew blood vessels, skin, and bone. More immediately, eating dark chocolate releases our beta-endorphins, or "happy chemicals."

- Caffeine and theobromine can boost energy and, in moderation, help to balance blood-sugar levels.
- Contains healthy monounsaturated fats, shown to keep the heart youthful and strong.

Practical tips:
The health benefits only apply to good-quality dark chocolate—the milk and sugar in milk chocolate negate these. Eating dark chocolate with at least 70 percent cocoa solids will raise your antioxidant levels. Remember that chocolate also has a high caffeine content—an average small bar of chocolate contains the equivalent amount of caffeine of one-third of a cup of coffee.

MOLE SAUCE

SERVES 6–8

9 mixed chiles, soaked in hot water for 30 minutes

1 onion, sliced

2–3 garlic cloves, crushed

½ cup sesame seeds

¾ cup toasted slivered almonds

1 teaspoon ground coriander

4 cloves

2–3 tablespoons olive oil

1½ cups chicken stock

4 tomatoes, chopped

2 teaspoons ground cinnamon

⅓ cup raisins

¾ cup pumpkin seeds

2 ounces dark chocolate

1 tablespoon red wine vinegar

METHOD

1 Drain the chiles and put into a blender with the onion, garlic, sesame seeds, almonds, coriander, and cloves and process to form a thick paste.

2 Heat the oil in a saucepan, add the paste, and cook for 5 minutes. Add the stock, tomatoes, cinnamon, raisins, and pumpkin seeds. Bring to a boil, reduce the heat, and simmer, stirring occasionally, for 15 minutes.

3 Break the chocolate into pieces and add to the sauce with the vinegar. Cook gently for 5 minutes, then use as required. It is usually served with poultry.

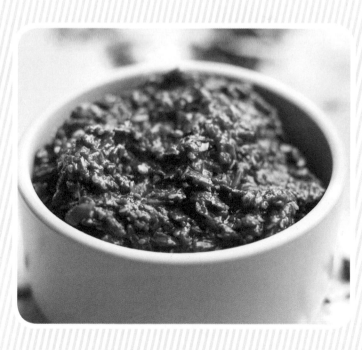

DARK CHOCOLATE ROULADE

SERVES 6–8

butter, for greasing

6 ounces semisweet dark chocolate, broken into squares

4 extra-large eggs, separated

½ cup granulated sugar

unsweetened cocoa powder, sifted, for dusting

8 ounces white chocolate, broken into squares

1 cup mascarpone cheese or heavy cream

raspberry coulis, to serve

METHOD

1   Preheat the oven to 350°F. Grease a 13 x 9-inch jelly-roll pan and line with parchment paper.

2   Melt the dark chocolate in a heatproof bowl set over a saucepan of simmering water, being careful that the bowl does not touch the water. Remove from the heat and let cool slightly.

3   Put the egg yolks and sugar into a bowl and beat until pale and thick. Beat the egg whites in a separate bowl until they hold soft peaks. Stir the melted chocolate into the egg yolk mixture, then fold in the beatened egg whites.

4   Spread the batter into the prepared pan. Bake in the preheated oven for 15–20 minutes, until risen and firm. Dust a sheet of parchment paper with cocoa powder. Turn out the roulade onto the paper, cover with a clean dish towel, and let cool.

5   Meanwhile, melt the white chocolate in a heatproof bowl set over a saucepan of simmering water, Remove from the heat and let cool slightly. Stir into the mascarpone cheese.

6   Uncover the roulade, remove the parchment paper, and spread with the white chocolate cream. Use the paper to roll up the roulade to enclose the filling. Serve with raspberry coulis.

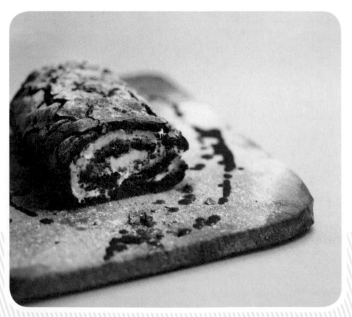

DARK CHOCOLATE & NUT COOKIES

MAKES 18

1⅔ cups all-purpose flour, plus extra for dusting

½ teaspoon baking soda

1 stick unsalted butter, chilled and diced, plus extra for greasing

⅔ cup firmly packed light brown sugar

2 tablespoons corn syrup

1 egg, beaten

⅓ cup blanched hazelnuts, chopped

½ cup chopped pecans

5 ouces semisweet chocolate, broken into pieces

METHOD

1 Preheat the oven to 375°F. Lightly grease two large baking sheets

2 Sift the flour and baking soda into a large bowl. Add the butter and rub it in with your fingertips until the mixture resembles fine bread crumbs. Stir in the sugar, syrup, egg, and two-thirds of the hazelnuts and pecans and mix thoroughly.

3 Drop tablespoonfuls of the dough onto the prepared baking sheets, spaced well apart. Flatten slightly with the back of the spoon and top with the remaining nuts.

4 Bake in the preheated oven for 7–9 minutes, or until golden brown. Let cool on the baking sheets for 5 minutes, then transfer to a wire rack to cool completely.

5 Melt the chocolate in a heatproof bowl set over a saucepan of simmering water. Dip the top of each cooled cookie in the chocolate, then let stand on a wire rack in a cool place until the chocolate has set.

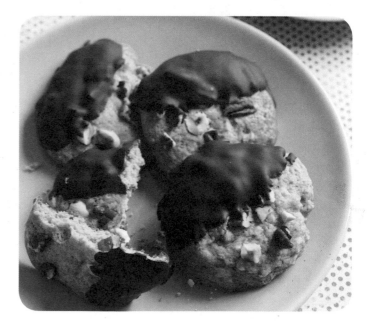

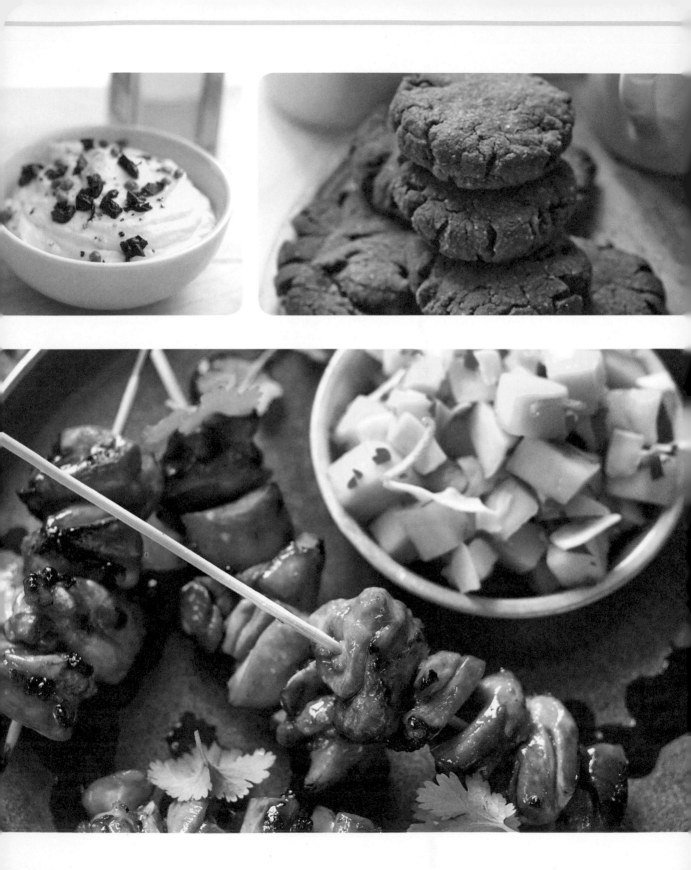

NUTS & OILS

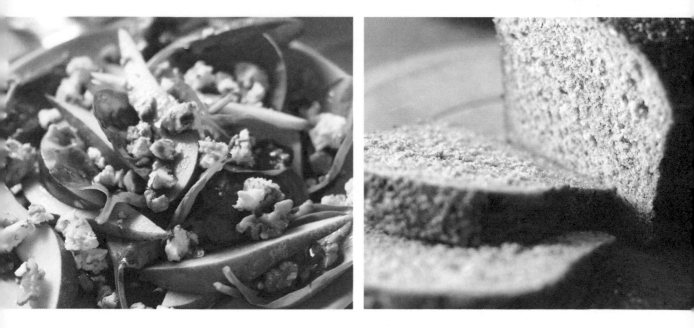

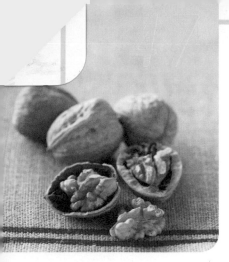

WALNUTS

Known for their unusually high content of omega-3 fats, the nutrients in walnuts can help prevent heart disease, cancers, arthritis, and common skin complaints.

MAJOR NUTRIENTS PER ¼ CUP/1¼ OUNCES WALNUTS

Calories	196
Total fat	19.5g
Protein	4.5g
Carbohydrate	4g
Fiber	2g
Niacin	0.3mg
Vitamin B6	0.16mg
Calcium	29mg
Potassium	132mg
Magnesium	47mg
Iron	0.9mg
Zinc	0.9mg

Unlike most nuts, walnuts are much richer in polyunsaturated fats than in monounsaturates. The type of polyunsaturates that walnuts contain is mostly the essential omega-3 fats, in the form of alpha-linolenic acid—just one portion will provide you with more than a day's recommended intake. An adequate and balanced intake of the omega fats has been linked with protection from cardiovascular disease, cancers, arthritis, skin problems, and diseases of the nervous system. For people who don't eat fish and fish oils, an intake of omega-3 fats from other sources, such as walnuts, flaxseeds, and soybeans, is important.

- Good source of fiber and the B vitamins.
- Rich in omega-3 fats and antioxidants.
- Good source of a range of important minerals.
- Can lower bad cholesterol and blood pressure and increase elasticity of the arteries.

Practical tips:
The high levels of polyunsaturated fats mean that walnuts spoil fairly quickly. Buy nuts with their shells on, if possible, store in the refrigerator, and consume quickly. Avoid buying chopped walnuts unless they are for immediate use—chopping speeds the oxidation of the nuts. Walnuts are best eaten raw as a snack, but they can also be added to cakes and other baked treats.

WALNUT & SEED BREAD

MAKES 2 LARGE LOAVES

3¾ cups whole-wheat flour

3⅓ cups white bread flour, plus extra for dusting

2 tablespoons sesame seeds

2 tablespoons sunflower seeds

2 tablespoons poppy seeds

1 cup whole walnuts, chopped

2 teaspoons salt

2 teaspoons active dry yeast

2 tablespoons olive oil or walnut oil

3 cups lukewarm water

1 tablespoon melted butter or oil, for greasing

METHOD

1   Mix together the flours, seeds, walnuts, salt, and yeast in a large bowl. Add the oil and water and stir well to form a soft dough. Invert the dough onto a lightly floured surface and knead well for 5–7 minutes, or until smooth and elastic.

2   Return the dough to the bowl, cover with a damp dish towel, and let stand in a warm place for 1–1½ hours to rise, or until the dough has doubled in size. Invert the dough onto a lightly floured surface and knead again for 1 minute.

3   Grease two 9-inch loaf pans with the butter. Divide the dough in half. Shape one piece to the length of the pan and three times the width. Fold the dough in three lengthwise and place in one of the pans with the seam underneath. Repeat with the other piece of dough. Cover and put in a warm place for about 30 minutes, or until the bread is well risen.

4   Meanwhile, preheat the oven to 450°F. Bake in the center of the preheated oven for 25–30 minutes, or until golden brown. Transfer to a wire rack to cool.

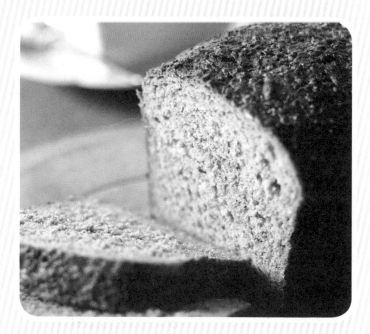

PINACH, PEAR & WALNUT SALAD

SERVES 2

3 cups baby leaf spinach

2 ripe pears, quartered, cored and thinly sliced

3 tablespoons chopped walnuts

½ cup crumbled soft blue cheese, to serve

DRESSING

1 tablespoon extra virgin olive oil

2 tablespoons balsamic vinegar

salt and pepper, to taste

METHOD

1   To make the dressing, put the olive oil and balsamic vinegar in a small bowl. Season with salt and pepper and whisk until thoroughly combined.

2   Put the spinach leaves into a salad bowl and add just enough of the dressing to coat the leaves lightly. Add the pears and the walnuts and toss to combine. Add the rest of the dressing, to taste. Serve with the cheese scattered on top.

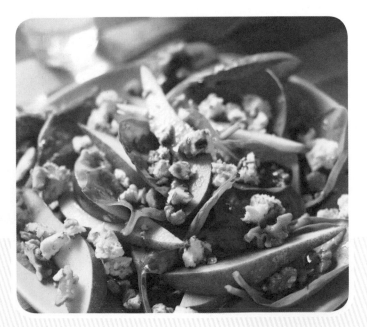

PUMPKIN & WALNUT CAKE

SERVES 12

1½ sticks butter,
plus extra for greasing

¾ cup firmly packed light
brown sugar

3 eggs, beaten

1 (15-ounce) can pumpkin
puree

1 teaspoon gluten-free
baking soda

3 tablespoons milk

4⅓ cups self-rising flour

1 teaspoon xanthan gum

½ teaspoon baking powder

¾ cup chopped walnuts

ICING

1¼ cups confectioners' sugar

pulp and juice of
2 passion fruit

2 teaspoons lime zest

METHOD

1   Preheat the oven to 350°F. Grease an 8-inch round springform cake pan and line with parchment paper.

2   Cream together the butter and sugar in a large bowl until fluffy. Stir in the eggs, slowly, one at a time, then stir in the pumpkin.

3   Add the baking soda to the milk and then add to the pumpkin mixture.

4   In a separate bowl, sift together the flour, xanthan gum, and baking powder and then fold the mixture into the pumpkin mixture with the walnuts.

5   Spoon the batter into the prepared cake pan and bake in the preheated oven for 40–45 minutes, until a toothpick inserted into the center comes out clean.

6   Remove from the oven and let cool in the pan for 10 minutes before transferring to a wire rack to cool completely.

7   To make the icing, sift the confectioners' sugar into a bowl and then add the passion fruit pulp and the lime zest. Stir well and pour over the cooled cake.

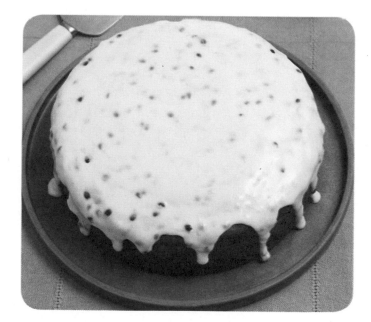

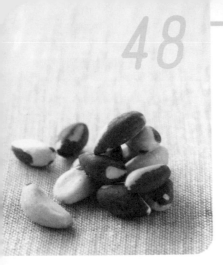

48

BRAZIL NUTS

One of the richest food sources of the antioxidant mineral selenium, Brazil nuts are also a good source of calcium and magnesium for healthy bones.

Brazil nuts have a high total fat content. Much of this is monounsaturated, but there is also a reasonable amount of polyunsaturates and high content of omega-6 linoleic acid, one of the essential fats. When cooked at high temperatures, these fats oxidize and are no longer healthy, so Brazil nuts are best eaten raw. The nut has an extremely high content of the mineral selenium and, on average, just one to two nuts can provide a whole day's recommended intake. Selenium is vital for the healthy function of internal organs, such as the liver, kidneys, and pancreas. Brazil nuts are also a good source of magnesium and calcium.

- Extremely rich in selenium, a mineral often lacking in modern diets.
- High magnesium content protects heart and bones.
- A good source of vitamin E for healthy skin and healing.

Practical tips:
Keep unshelled nuts in a cool, dry, dark place for up to six months. Shelled nuts should be stored in the refrigerator and consumed within a few weeks because their high fat content means they spoil quickly. They are best eaten raw.

MAJOR NUTRIENTS PER ¼ CUP/1¼ OUNCES BRAZIL NUTS

Calories	197
Total fat	19.9g
Protein	4.3g
Carbohydrate	3.7g
Fiber	2.3g
Vitamin E	1.7mcg
Calcium	48mg
Potassium	198mg
Magnesium	113mg
Zinc	1.2mg
Selenium	575mcg

DID YOU KNOW?

Brazil nuts are not actually nuts, but seeds that are enclosed in a hard fruit. The trees grow wild in the Amazon rain forests of Brazil and are rarely successfully cultivated.

TRAIL MIX

MAKES 12 SERVINGS

⅔ cup chopped dried apricots
½ cup dried cranberries
¾ cup roasted cashew nuts
⅔ cup shelled hazelnuts
⅔ cup shelled Brazil nuts, halved
¾ cup slivered almonds
¼ cup toasted pumpkin seeds
¼ cup sunflower seeds
¼ cup toasted pine nuts

METHOD

1   Place all the ingredients in an airtight container, close the lid, and shake several times. Shake the container before each opening, then reseal. This mix will stay fresh for up to two weeks if tightly sealed after each opening.

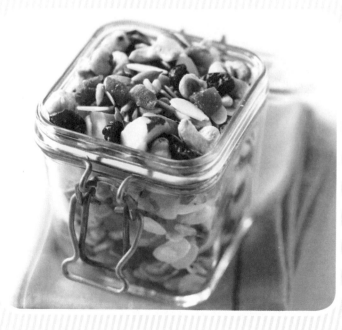

CHUNKY LENTIL & BRAZIL NUT ROAST

SERVES 6

margarine, for greasing

1 cup red lentils (available in health-food stores)

1 bay leaf

2 tablespoons olive oil

1 onion, finely chopped

2 garlic cloves, finely chopped

1 carrot, finely chopped

2 cups Brazil nuts

1 tablespoon tomato paste

1 tablespoon soy sauce

3 cups fresh white vegan bread crumbs

1 tablespoon dried oregano

steamed green vegetables, to serve

METHOD

1   Preheat the oven to 375°F. Grease and line a 9-inch loaf pan.

2   Put the lentils and bay leaf in a large saucepan with 1½ cups of water. Bring to a boil and then simmer for 25 minutes, or until the lentils are cooked to a mush. Remove and discard the bay leaf and set aside.

3   Heat the oil in a large skillet over medium heat. Sauté the onion, garlic, and carrot for 3 minutes. Coarsely chop one-third of the Brazil nuts. Place the remaining nuts in a food processor and pulse until processed to a powder. Transfer the onion mixture to a large mixing bowl with the ground and chopped nuts, lentils, tomato paste, soy sauce, bread crumbs, and oregano. Mix thoroughly and press into the prepared pan.

4   Bake in the preheated oven for 25 minutes. Let cool a little in the pan before turning out and slicing. Serve hot or cold with steamed green vegetables.

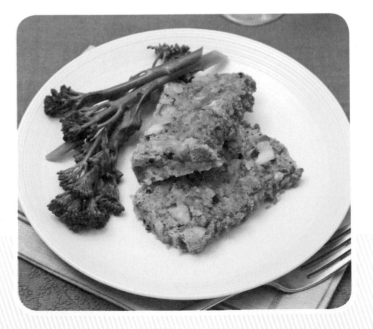

CHOCOLATE & BRAZIL NUT CRUNCHIES

MAKES 30

4 tablespoons butter or margarine, plus extra for greasing

¼ cup vegetable shortening

¾ cup raw brown sugar

1 egg

1 teaspoon vanilla extract

1 tablespoon milk

¾ cup all-purpose flour

1 cup rolled oats

1 teaspoon baking soda

pinch of salt

1 cup semisweet chocolate chips

½ cup Brazil nuts, chopped

METHOD

1 Put the butter, shortening, sugar, egg, vanilla extract, and milk in a blender or food processor and process for at least 3 minutes, until a fluffy consistency is reached.

2 Mix together the flour, oats, baking soda, and salt in a large bowl. Stir in the egg mixture, then the chocolate chips and nuts, and mix well together. Cover the bowl with plastic wrap and chill in the refrigerator for 30 minutes, until firm.

3 Meanwhile, preheat the oven to 350°F. Grease a large baking sheet.

4 Put 30 rounded tablespoonfuls of the dough onto the prepared baking sheet, making sure that they are well spaced. Bake in the preheated oven for 15 minutes, or until golden brown.

5 Transfer to a wire rack to cool before serving.

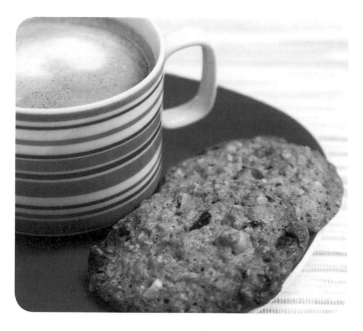

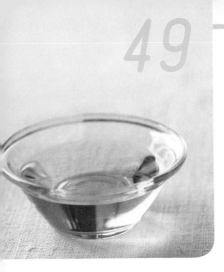

49

COCONUT OIL

Cooking with coconut oil is a simple way to reduce your exposure to the aging free radicals that are produced when roasting, frying, and baking.

MAJOR NUTRIENTS PER 1 TABLESPOON COCONUT OIL

Calories	129
Total fat	15g
Lauric acid	6.69g
Caprylic acid	1.125g
Myristic acid	2.5g
Omega-6 oils	270mg
Omega-9 oils	870mg
Protein	Trace
Carbohydrate	Trace
Fiber	Trace

Whenever we cook with oil, the heat causes damage to the oil's fat molecules, which has a knock-on effect when ingested. The free radicals produced can damage tissues and make us more susceptible to cancer, heart disease, and osteoporosis. Of all the saturated fats, coconut oil is the least prone to damage by heat, light, and oxygen, and can be heated to temperatures as high as 375°F. Coconut oil contains about 60 percent medium-chain triglycerides (MCTs), plant-based oils that raise metabolism and cannot be stored as fat in our bodies.

• The fats in coconut oil help renew the lining of the digestive tract, making sure of good digestion.
• Regular consumption has been shown to assist thyroid function and regulate metabolism and mood.

Practical tips:
Coconut oil, which becomes a clear liquid when heated, can be used in all kinds of cooking and doesn't retain any of the coconut flavor from the flesh. It does behave differently from other oils, however, so a little experimentation may be necessary. Choose an unprocessed variety, and avoid any that have been hydrogenated or contain preservatives.

THAI GREEN CURRY

SERVES 4

2 tablespoons coconut oil

2 tablespoons Thai green curry paste

1 pound skinless, boneless chicken breasts, cut into cubes

2 kaffir lime leaves, coarsely torn

1 lemongrass stalk, finely chopped

1 cup canned coconut milk

16 baby eggplants, halved

2 tablespoons Thai fish sauce

fresh Thai basil sprigs and thinly sliced kaffir lime leaves, to garnish

METHOD

1 Heat a large wok or skillet over medium heat. Add the oil and heat for 30 seconds. Add the Thai curry paste and stir-fry briefly until all the aromas are released.

2 Add the chicken, lime leaves, and lemongrass and stir-fry for 3–4 minutes, until the meat is beginning to brown. Add the coconut milk and eggplants and simmer gently for 8–10 minutes, or until tender.

3 Stir in the fish sauce and serve immediately, garnished with Thai basil sprigs and lime leaves.

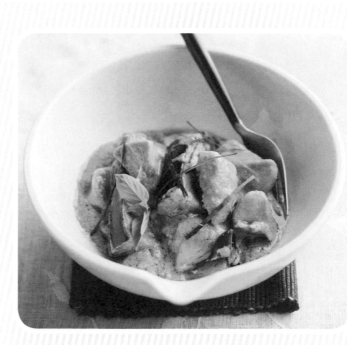

COCONUT & LIME CHICKEN

SERVES 2

2 tablespoons coconut oil, melted and cooled

zest and juice of 1 lime, plus extra wedges for serving

2 tablespoons soy sauce

1 tablespoon brown sugar

4 skinless boneless chicken thighs, any excess fat removed, sliced into pieces

salt, to taste

MANGO SALSA

1 ripe mango, peeled and flesh diced

1 small red chile, seeded and finely diced

juice and zest of ½ lime

small bunch of coriander, leaves chopped

handful toasted coconut flakes

METHOD

1 In a bowl mix the lime, soy, and sugar. Add the chicken pieces stirring to coat, then set aside to marinade for 1 hour (or 30 minutes if short of time). Stir in the coconut oil.

2 For the salsa, combine all of the ingredients. Cover and set to one side for the flavors to mingle. Preheat the broiler to medium-high. If using wooden skewers, soak them in water for 20 minutes

3 Thread the chicken pieces onto the skewers and season with salt. Pour any leftover marinade into a small saucepan and bubble for a couple of minutes until thickened.

4 Place the skewers onto a wire rack with a tray underneath. Cook under the preheated broiler for 10–12 minutes, turning halfway, and basting occasionally with the marinade, until golden, sticky, and cooked through. Drizzle the skewers with any leftover marinade, and serve with the mango salsa and extra lime wedges for squeezing.

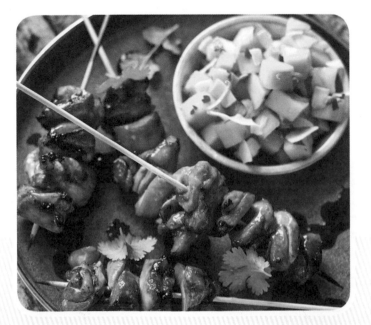

VEGAN CHOC CHIP COOKIES

MAKES 24

¹⁄₃ cup coconut oil, melted and cooled

½ cup lightly packed soft light brown sugar

2 tablespoons soya milk

1 teaspoon vanilla extract

1 cup plus 1 tablespoon all-purpose flour

1 cup almond meal (ground almonds)

2 tablespoons vegan cocoa powder

1 teaspoon baking powder

pinch of salt

2¼ ounces vegan semi-sweet chocolate, roughly chopped

METHOD

1   Preheat the oven to 350°F, and line a large cookie sheet with baking paper. Put the coconut oil and sugar into a large bowl and beat with an electric whisk for 5 minutes, or until pale and creamy. Add the milk and vanilla.

2   Mix the flour, almond meal, cocoa, baking powder, and salt together. Tip into the bowl and stir until well combined. Add the chopped chocolate, mixing until evenly distributed.

3   Roll the dough into 24 balls and place on the prepared cookie sheet, spaced well apart. Flatten slightly with the palm of your hand. Put into the oven to bake for 12 minutes, or until firm around the edges but still a little soft in the center. Remove and allow to cool for 5 minutes on the cookie sheet before transferring to a wire rack to cool.

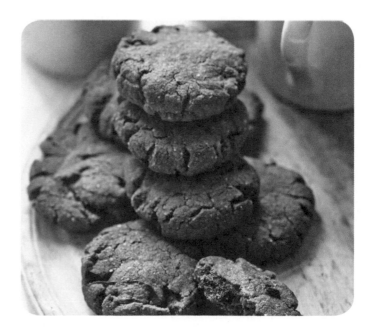

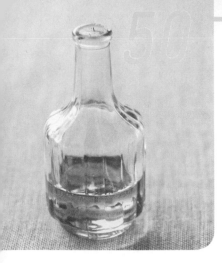

OLIVE OIL

Well known for being high in heart-protective monounsaturates, virgin olive oils also contain a range of antioxidant plant compounds and vitamin E.

MAJOR NUTRIENTS PER 1 TABLESPOON OLIVE OIL

Calories	130
Total fat	15g
Protein	Trace
Carbohydrate	Trace
Fiber	Trace
Vitamin C	Trace
Potassium	Trace
Lycopene	Trace
Lutein/Zeaxanthin	Trace

The main type of fat in olive oil is monounsaturated, which helps prevent cholesterol from being deposited on artery walls and, therefore, helps protect us from cardiovascular disease and strokes. In addition, early pressings of the olives (as in extra virgin olive oil, particularly "cold-pressed" oil) produce an oil that is rich in beneficial plant compounds. These can protect against cancer and high blood pressure, and they can lower cholesterol and the compound oleocanthal, an anti-inflammatory with similar action to ibuprofen. Finally, olive oil is a good source of vitamin E.

• Helps improve blood cholesterol profile and protect us from cardiovascular disease.
• Rich in polyphenols to protect against colon and other cancers.
• Can help prevent *H. pylori*, which can lead to stomach ulcers.
• Antibacterial and antioxidant.

Practical tips:
Olive oil should be stored in the dark and used within two months of opening. When buying olive oil, choose a store that keeps it in dimly lit conditions and has high turnover. For the full benefit of olive oil, eat it cold in salad dressings or drizzled on bread or vegetables. Don't use extra virgin olive oil for cooking at high temperatures or the beneficial chemicals will be destroyed.

DID YOU KNOW?

Light destroys many of the disease-fighting compounds in olive oil; after a year, oils stored in clear bottles under store lighting have shown at least a 30 percent decrease in antioxidants.

BASIL OIL

MAKES 1 CUP

2 cups fresh basil leaves
2 cloves garlic, halved
1 cup olive oil

METHOD

1   Wash the basil leaves and dry them well. Prepare a bowl of ice water.

2   Bring a saucepan of water to a boil, add the basil leaves, and blanch for five seconds. Scoop out the leaves and plunge immediately into the ice water to stop the cooking process. Drain out all the water and squeeze the leaves to get rid of as much of the water as possible. Dry them between layers of paper towels. Chop coarsely and place in a clean jar. Add the garlic.

3   Gently heat the oil over low heat until warmed and fragrant—about five minutes. Be sure that it does not boil or burn. Remove from the heat and pour the oil into a clean jar over the basil leaves. Let cool, cover, and store in the refrigerator. Strain out the basil within a week.

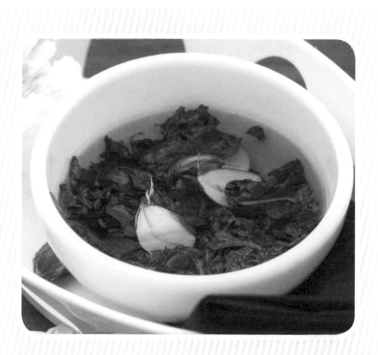

TARAMASALATA

SERVES 6

8 ounces smoked cod roe
1 small onion, quartered
1 cup fresh white bread crumbs
1 large garlic clove, crushed
grated rind and juice of 1 large lemon
⅔ cup extra virgin olive oil
6 tablespoons hot water
pepper, to taste
black olives and capers, to garnish

METHOD

1   Remove the skin from the fish roe. Put the onion in a food processor and chop finely. Add the cod roe in small pieces and process until smooth. Add the bread crumbs, garlic, lemon rind and juice, and mix well together.

2   With the machine running, very slowly pour in the oil. When all the oil has been added, blend in the water. Season with pepper.

3   Transfer the mixture to a serving bowl and chill in the refrigerator for at least 1 hour before serving. Serve garnished with olives and capers.

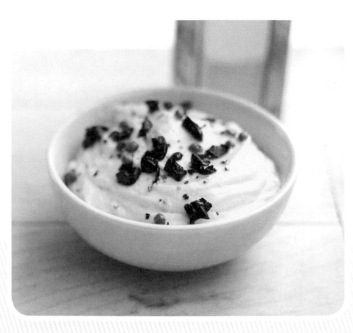

TAGLIATELLE WITH PESTO

SERVES 4

1 pound dried tagliatelle

salt

fresh basil sprigs, to garnish

PESTO

2 garlic cloves

¼ cup pine nuts

1¼ cups fresh basil leaves

½ cup olive oil

½ cup freshly grated
Parmesan-style vegetarian
cheese

salt, to taste

METHOD

1 To make the pesto, put the garlic, pine nuts, and salt into a food processor or blender and process briefly. Add the basil leaves and process to a paste. With the motor still running, gradually add the oil. Scrape into a bowl and beat in the cheese. Season to taste with salt.

2 Bring a large, heavy saucepan of lightly salted water to a boil. Add the pasta, return to a boil, and cook for 8–10 minutes, or until tender but still firm to the bite. Drain the pasta well, return to the pan, and toss with half of the pesto, then divide among warmed serving dishes and top with the remaining pesto. Garnish with basil and serve immediately.

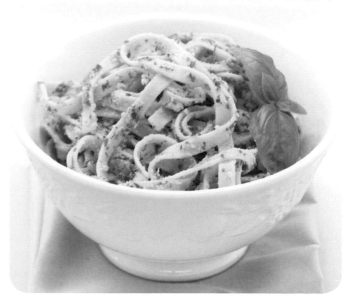

INDEX

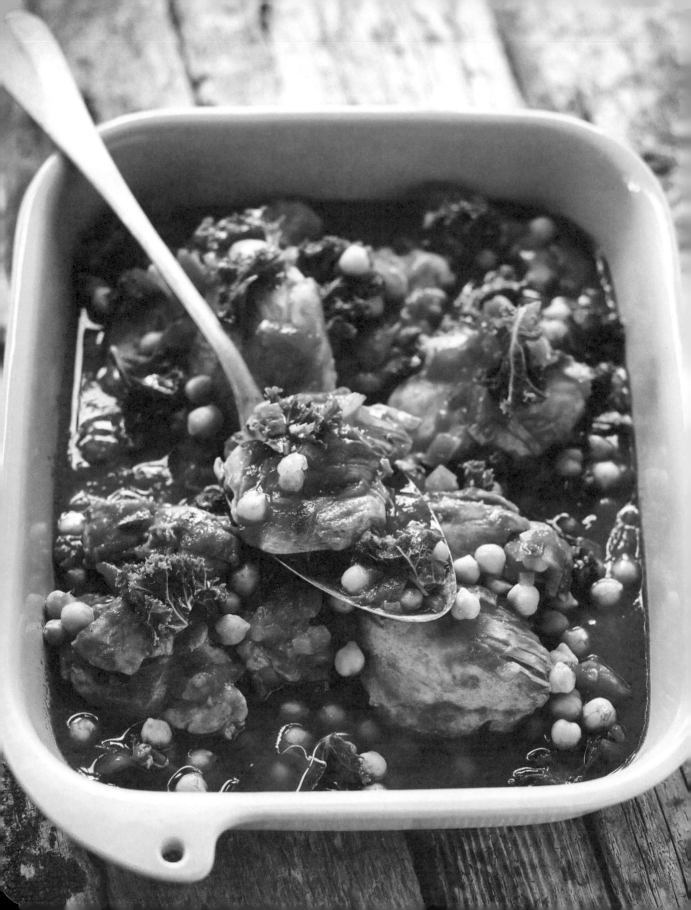